Osteoporosis: A Clinical Guide

Second Edition

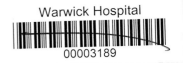

Osteoporosis:
A Clinical Guide

Second Edition

Anthony D Woolf BSc FRCP

Consultant Rheumatologist, Royal Cornwall Hospital, Truro

Allan St John Dixon MD FRCP

Honorary Consultant Physician, Royal United Hospital and
Royal National Hospital for Rheumatic Diseases, Bath

MARTIN DUNITZ

First published in the United Kingdom in 1998 by
Martin Dunitz Ltd
The Livery House
7–9 Pratt Street
London NW1 0AE

A CIP catalogue record for this book is available from the British Library.

ISBN 1–85317–246–4

Distributed in the United States by:
Blackwell Science Inc.
Commerce Place, 350 Main Street
Malden, MA 02148, USA
Tel: 1-800-215-1000

Distributed in Canada by:
Login Brothers Book Company
324 Salteaux Crescent
Winnipeg, Manitoba, R3J 3T2
Canada
Tel: 204-224-4068

Distributed in Brazil by:
Ernesto Reichmann Distribuidora de Livros, Ltda
Rua Coronel Marques 335, Tatuape 03440-000
Sao Paulo,
Brazil

Composition by Scribe Design, Gillingham, Kent, United Kingdom
Printed and bound in Spain by Grafos, S.A.

Contents

Preface to the second edition

The first edition of this book was published in 1988. Since then, knowledge of osteoporosis has increased greatly but there are still many problems not yet solved. Medical audit has become widespread and there is emphasis on evidence-based clinical practice. What is known and what needs to be known will be emphasized.

Osteoporosis has been more clearly defined and the impact in terms of morbidity, mortality and socioeconomic costs is recognized everywhere. There is more awareness of osteoporosis at public, professional and political levels and calls for preventive strategies. Prevention, however, implies prediction. The prediction of risk and the identification of those most likely to be at risk have also made significant advances. Best practice in gynaecology includes taking responsibility to ensure that women who have had a bilateral oophorectomy should be treated with hormone replacement therapy. The same applies to women who, for whatever reason, prematurely lose their normal levels of circulating oestrogens. Best practice in orthopaedic and fracture clinics means that older subjects presenting with *any* fracture should be regarded as at risk of later, more serious osteoporosis-related fractures and appropriate referrals made, usually, and where available, to a specialized osteoporosis unit. Prevention in childhood and young adult life has been

recognized as vital and research has proved the importance of exercise and a high calcium diet in these age groups. Good bones built up during the phase of bone growth will resist the inevitable loss of bone mineral in the later years. There has been more knowledge of the hereditability of osteoporosis and some of the contributing genes have been identified.

Nearly all economically advanced countries now have specialist scientific societies to tackle the problem and most of them also have 'self-help' societies to support those with osteoporosis. The specialist scientific journal *Osteoporosis International* is now well established. International epidemiological studies at the European level have been successfully undertaken. Hormone replacement therapy (HRT) is accepted as the gold standard for prevention of osteoporosis in women and in this cardiologists have become professional allies, as HRT is second in importance only to stopping smoking in strategies for the prevention of cardiovascular disease in women.

There have been technical improvements in devices for measuring bone density, giving negligible radiation exposure, rapid results and better methods of identifying those at high risk and of following the results of treatments. Bone formation and breakdown can be assessed with markers of extraordinary sensitivity and specificity. Treatments have become available to prevent further fractures in established osteoporosis. The bisphosphonates have been shown to be potent treatments for secondary prevention of osteoporosis. New forms of HRT deliver 'no-bleed' treatment without loss of protection against endometrial cancer and selective oestrogen receptor modulators are being developed to target the skeleton. Calcitonin has analgesic effects as well as protective effects in spinal osteoporosis. Specialist geriatric rehabilitation units reduce mortality and dependency after osteoporotic hip fractures.

But there have also been failures in advancement. Fluoride, which reliably increases bone mineral density, has fallen out of favour because it may increase bone brittleness. We still have not teased out an anatomical answer to the question as to why some spinal osteoporosis sufferers have little or no pain when others have their lives made miserable by severe and enduring pain. There have been no advances in finding the cause of generalized idiopathic osteoporosis in juveniles, in young men, in women before the menopause or in some women in association with pregnancy. There is evidence from studies of their actions on the cardiovascular system that the various oestrogens have qualitatively different effects, but we do not yet know if this applies to their use in female osteoporosis. In humans, and in physically active animals, prolonged immobilization leads rapidly to osteoporosis, but we do not know why it does not do so in bears, which hibernate in the long subarctic winter. In murine and turkey models of experimental osteoporosis, certain kinds of pulsed electromagnetic radiation have been shown to prevent loss of calcium from the bones. This has lead to the promotion of bogus black-box treatments claiming to cure existing osteoporosis in the human without any evidence that would pass critical peer review.

Another failure, only slowly being addressed, is the sometimes scandalous management of elderly people brought to hospital for an osteoporotic fracture of the hip. This was identified in a Royal College of Physicians report in 1989.

There is still much to be done.

1 Physiological background

INTRODUCTION

Bone is an organ that gives form to the body, supporting its weight, protecting vital organs, and facilitating locomotion by providing attachments for muscles to act as levers.

Bone is also a special mineralized tissue, which, like reinforced concrete, is a 'composite' in materials science terms—a meshwork of collagen fibres embedded in a matrix of minerals. Despite its hardness, it is metabolically active, continually being formed and resorbed by bone cells whose activity is modified by many factors. It grows, maintaining approximately the same shape from birth to maturity, but can respond to physical forces at any age and if broken will repair itself as nearly as possible to the original shape. Bone is also an ion reservoir containing over 99% of the total body calcium. Its role in this respect is of vital importance.

STRUCTURE OF BONE

Organization of bone

Macroscopic anatomy

Bones can be conveniently divided into flat bones such as the scapula, skull and pelvis, and tubular bones, which include the limb bones and vertebral bodies. The dense outer surface or cortex is composed of compact bone and the centre or medulla is braced by narrow plates or trabeculae, a construction which endows the maximum strength for the minimum weight. In the interstices of the medulla lies the bone marrow, where bone cells are in close contact with haemopoietic cells. In infancy the marrow is red but in adults this retreats to the bone ends, to be replaced by yellow or fatty marrow.

A typical tubular bone has a central diaphysis or shaft, a metaphysis and an epiphysis capped with the articular cartilage at each end (Figure 1.1). Tubular bones grow in length by ossification at the metaphysis at cartilage growth plates (endochondral ossification). The cortex grows in diameter by subperiosteal deposition accompanied by endosteal resorption. This process leads to enlargement of the marrow cavity. Flat bones develop by intramembranous bone formation.

An ossifying growth plate can be divided into functional zones (Figure 1.2). Chondrocytes initially proliferate and then actively synthesize matrix, the cells having an internal arrangement typical of secretory cells. Next, the cells hypertrophy, compressing the surrounding matrix. In the next zone calcification is found, initially with small isolated clusters of crystals, which then coalesce to an almost solid mass at the cartilage–bone junction. Capillary buds, osteoprogenitor cells and osteoclasts then penetrate

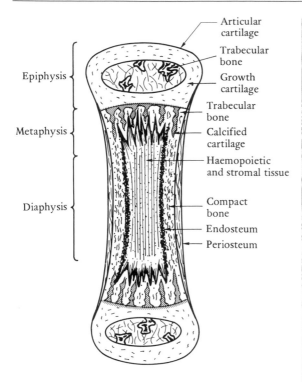

Figure 1.1 Structure of a tubular bone. In an immature bone primary ossification centres in the diaphysis move progressively towards the bone ends. In most tubular bones there are also secondary ossification centres in the epiphyses. A cartilaginous growth plate remains between these ossification centres until growth ceases. The distal remnant of cartilage becomes the articulating surface. Throughout growth the cartilage growth plate maintains an almost constant thickness, but at a set age for each bone the growth plate becomes ossified with fusion of the epiphyses to the diaphysis.

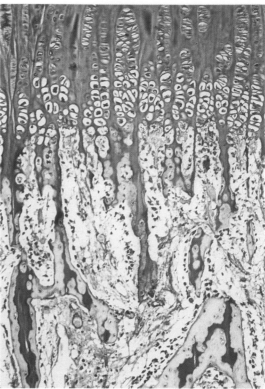

Figure 1.2 The growth plate of a rat long bone showing the proliferating zone at the top, with matrix synthesis below, and calcification of matrix at the bottom.

and resorb this somewhat amorphous mineralized matrix and new bone formed by the osteoblasts replaces it.

Microscopic anatomy

Compact bone

Compact or cortical bone constitutes 80% of the skeletal mass. It forms the outer surface of all bone but the majority is found in the shafts of tubular bone.

Compact bone is composed of lamellae, which are concentrically arranged around a small central canal to form a Haversian system or osteon (see Figure 1.3). Between the lamellae are osteocytes lying in lacunae, which are connected with each other and with the central canal by fine canaliculi. Osteocytes lie no more than 300 μm from a blood vessel; the average cross-sectional diameter of a Haversian system is 500 μm. The Haversian systems, which may be up to 5 mm long, run parallel to the long

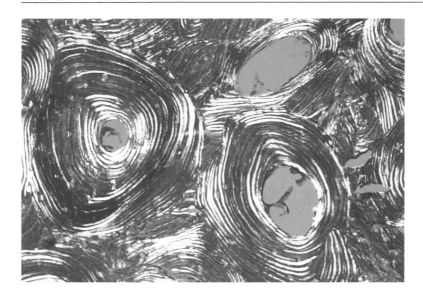

Figure 1.3 A reticulin stain of cortical bone showing the Haversian systems.

axis of the bone, branching and communicating with each other. There are also interstitial lamellae between the Haversian systems, and circumferential lamellae which encircle the inner and outer surface of the bone.

Periosteal vessels penetrate compact bone through nutrient canals in order to supply the marrow, and branches of these form the intracortical vessels that lie, along with the venules, within the Haversian canals. The interconnecting canaliculi between the osteocytes allow for rapid movement of fluid for their nutrition and humoral intercommunication.

Haversian systems are formed either by the deposition of new bone on the endosteal or periosteal surfaces of cortical bone (primary osteons), or by osteoclasts cutting tunnels (cutting cones) into bone with subsequent deposition of new bone by osteoblasts (secondary osteons). The latter process is found in bone that is remodelling itself, and the outer limit of a secondary osteon can be identified by a cement line which separates it from adjacent bone.

Trabecular bone

This is a rigid meshwork of mineralized bone which forms the greater part of each vertebral body and the epiphyses of the long bones, and is present at other sites such as the iliac crest. It contributes 20% of the total skeletal mass.

Complete struts are called trabeculae, but incomplete spicules are also seen (see Figure 1.4). The trabeculae usually lie so as to resist deformational stresses (either from weight bearing or from muscle activity) and their number, size and distribution are related to these forces. Trabecular bone provides a large surface area and is the most metabolically active part of the skeleton, with a high rate of turnover and a blood supply that is much greater than that of compact bone. It also acts as a calcium reservoir.

Trabeculae have a lamella arrangement of bone but are seldom thick enough to contain osteocytes. Growth occurs on their surfaces, which are covered by a layer of osteoid (that is, unmineralized matrix), which is produced

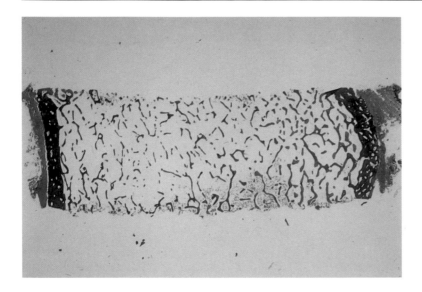

Figure 1.4   A section of normal bone showing both cortices of compact bone with medullary trabecular bone in between.

and subsequently mineralized by surface osteoblasts. Occasional osteoclasts lie on their surfaces in shallow pits known as Howship's lacunae.

Bone cells

Improved methods of preparing sections of bone for microscopic examination have made it apparent that cells cover the whole surface of bone and also lie within the lacunae. Most are mature osteoblasts or osteoclasts, others are osteocytes and lining cells. Yet other cell types that are found in contact with these cells on the surfaces of bone include bone progenitor cells and macrophages and mature and stem cells of the haemopoietic series (Figure 1.5 shows the various types of bone cells). Nor should one forget the fat cells which constitute most of the bone marrow in adult bones. Fat cells share a common lineage with osteocytes in the development of the embryo. There is much scope for cell–cell interaction.

Osteoblasts

Osteoblasts (see Figure 1.6) are the bone-forming cells. They synthesize bone matrix and are involved in its subsequent mineralization. They are usually seen as a single layer of cuboidal cells directly applied to the internal surfaces of bone. They are secretory cells, having a large Golgi zone and abundant rough endoplasmic reticulum. There are scattered mitochondria and attached to some of which are small granular mineral deposits composed of calcium, phosphate, a trace of magnesium and some organic matter. Mitochondria can remove calcium from the cell cytoplasm and deposit it in these granules, thus controlling intracellular calcium concentration. Microtubules are most abundant in cell processes and may be important in the flow of water, electrolytes and other intracellular substances. Contractile microfilaments provide the cell with an internal cytoskeleton and also give the cell motility.

The inactive osteoblast is a thin cell which may look more like a fibrocyte. Its cytoplasm

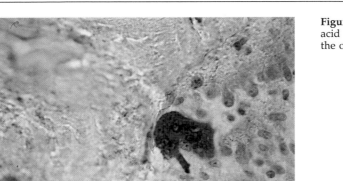

Figure 1.5 Bone cells. An acid phosphatase stain shows the osteoclasts as dark red.

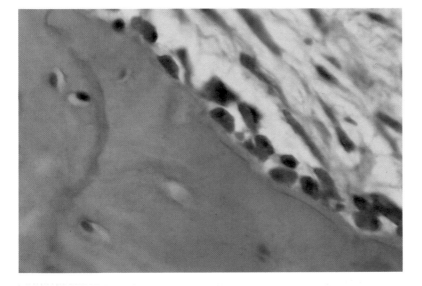

Figure 1.6 Osteoblasts applied to the bone surface.

may only just be apparent on ordinary microscopy. Changes in osteoblast morphology and activity are induced by calcium-regulating hormones and various growth factors. Bone-specific alkaline phosphatase is localized to the plasma membrane, and is present in large amounts. It has a role in bone formation but the exact mechanisms are unclear.

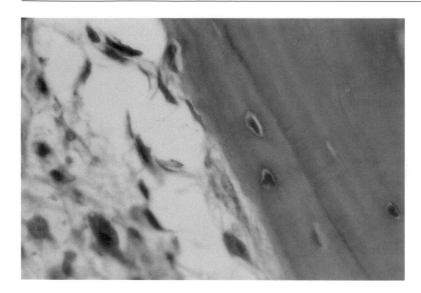

Figure 1.7　Osteocytes covering the bone surface as a flattened layer of cells.

Although the osteoblasts are closely applied to bone, their other surfaces are in contact with other cells, including osteoprogenitor cells. The proximity of these cells allows for interaction either by direct cell contact or by the release of cytokines.

Osteoblasts synthesize and secrete Type I collagen and mucopolysaccharides to form the bone matrix, which is laid down as a thin layer of osteoid between the osteoblasts and the calcification front. It is subsequently mineralized. In addition, they synthesize collagenase, prostaglandin E_2 (PGE$_2$) and the bone-associated proteins, osteocalcin and osteonectin. They have receptors to parathyroid hormone (PTH), calcitonin, calcitriol, PGE$_2$, glucocorticosteroids, interleukins-1α and 1β, and various cytokines.

The osteocyte (see Figure 1.7) is derived from the osteoblast. It either lies on the surface of bone or is encased within lacunae in mineralized bone, having surrounded itself with osteoid that has subsequently mineralized. Osteocytes are relatively inactive, but they show changes with PTH and calcitonin and may play a role in maintaining constant levels of calcium in the body fluids.

Osteoclasts

Osteoclasts (see Figure 1.8) are multinucleate cells that resorb calcified bone or cartilage. Macrophages can also resorb bone but this activity appears to be restricted to dead bone, whereas osteoclasts can resorb vital bone. They are derived from a stem cell of the monocyte/macrophage lineage. The early stages circulate in the blood as undifferentiated promonocytes—some of which attach to bone and develop into osteoclasts, losing some of their monocytic surface cell markers in the process. The mature osteoclasts have between two and 100 nuclei and measure from 200 to 200 000 μm^2 as a result of fusion of single nucleated cells which are difficult to identify in sections of bone.

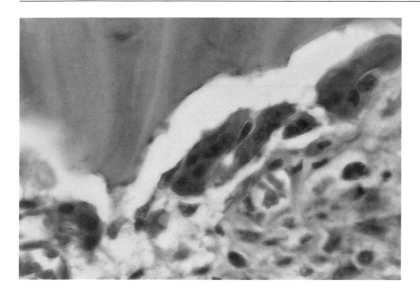

Figure 1.8 Osteoclasts and Howship's lacunae. The cells have become detached from the bone surface during fixation and decalcification.

Osteoclasts lie on bone surfaces or in pits (Howship's lacunae) where they have resorbed bone. The cell surface that is applied to bone, and at which active resorption occurs, appears ruffled. This is caused by the hundreds of motile microvilli directed at the resorbing surface. This area is sealed off from neighbouring cells to form a micro-environment adjacent to the mineralized bone. Osteoclast precursors proliferate in response to PTH, vitamin D or prostaglandins and either directly or through some intermediary mechanism are stimulated to secrete demineralizing acid and calcium-chelating anions (such as citrate) into this micro-environment. They also contain digestive vacuoles and vesicles and secrete acid hydrolases and neutral proteases to degrade matrix following demineralization. The probable role of collagenase, which is secreted by osteoblasts, is to remove surface protein and allow osteoclast attachment, with the help of adhesion molecules or integrins. It appears that most factors that activate osteoclasts act indirectly via osteoblasts: for instance, there are no receptors for 1,25-dihydroxy-vitamin D_3 on osteoclast surfaces, and PTH has in fact been shown to act in this way. The nature of the second messenger coupling osteoblastic to osteoclastic activity is uncertain.

The osteoclast is a very efficient cell. In bone which is actively remodelling there are six times as many osteoblasts as osteoclasts. Osteoclasts are mobile cells and after eroding one pit in mineralized bone may move to another site.

Bone matrix

Bone matrix comprises collagen and mucopolysaccharides and is mineralized. The mineral phase gives compressive strength and rigidity but it is the fibrous organic matrix that gives bone its resistance to tractional and torsional forces. The strength to weight ratio of bone is related to this integrated composition of collagen and mineral as well as to the microscopic arrangement of collagen fibres within the bone.

Organic matrix

Collagen is the main extracellular protein in the body and forms more than 25% of bone. It constitutes 65% of the total organic component of bone tissue. Bone cells, proteoglycans and lipids make up the rest.

Collagens in bone

Collagen consists of a helix of three long polypeptide chains, the alpha chains. The 13 or more main types of human collagen can be broadly categorized into fibrillar (Types I, II, III and V) and nonfibrillar (Table 1.1). Fibrillar collagens are the most abundant forms and are found in connective tissues throughout the body. Type I is overwhelmingly predominant in bone and also in skin and tendon. But bone is a complex tissue and in it there are small amounts of other collagens associated with cell basement membranes and the adventitia of blood vessels and capillaries in bone. Different collagens have different alpha chains, each related to a specific gene. Type I collagen is composed of two $\alpha 1(I)$ and one $\alpha 2(I)$ chains. The *COL1A1* gene is on chromosone 17 and the *COL1A2* gene is on chromosone 7.

The formation of collagen (Figure 1.9) occurs in steps. A protocollagen molecule is first synthesized. A number of post-translational modifications follow. In all, over 100 amino acids are modified in each pro-alpha chain. The principal modifications within the osteoblast are the hydroxylation of proline and lysine to form hydroxyproline and hydroxylysine. The alpha chains then form a triple helix before secretion. The C- and N-terminal propeptides are cleaved following secretion and in the final conversion of procollagen to collagen one-third of the mass is cleaved from the protein. The tropocollagen molecules self-

assemble into collagen fibrils. The basic triple helix structure is retained as the backbone of the molecule, strengthened by covalent cross-links which form during the maturation of collagen. Cross-links which contain both pyridinoline and deoxypyridinoline occur mainly at the C- and N-terminal parts of the collagen molecule where the triple helix is replaced by nontriple domains or telopeptides. In the turnover of collagen pyridinoline (Pyd) and deoxypyridinoline (Dpd) or the peptides which contain them are released from the terminal domains into the urine. The measurement and ratio of these breakdown products provide an index of bone resorption as these cross-links are only found in mature collagen. These markers are now widely employed as a way of assessing bone turnover and the effects of treatment.

On electron microscopy, collagen fibres have a distinct pattern of bands because of the staggered arrangement of the parallel tropocollagen molecules, with a gap between their ends (see Figure 1.9). Scanning electron

Table 1.1		Types of collagen	
Type	*Genetic data*	*Molecular formula*	*Tissue*
I	COL1A1 COL1A2	$\alpha 1(I)_2 \alpha 2(I)$	Major type in many tissues: bone, dentine, skin, tendon, blood vessel wall, gastrointestinal tract
II	COL2A1	$[\alpha 1(II)]_3$	Cartilage, vitreous humor, vertebral disc
III	COL3A1	$[\alpha 1(III)]_3$	Fetal tissues, with Type I in all tissues
V	COL5A1 COL5A2 COL5A3	$[\alpha 1(V)_2 \alpha(V)]_2$ and other forms	Vascular tissues and smooth muscle

Altogether, at least 14 differently structured collagens are known. Less common are Types VI to XIV, which are classed as nonfibrillar and have specialized functions and distribution. Some occur in bone associated with blood vessels and basement membranes.

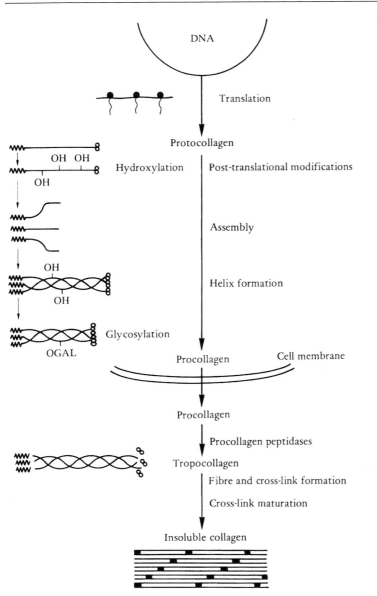

Figure 1.9   Biosynthesis of collagen.

microscopy shows a branching, interconnecting, intricately woven pattern of parallel collagen fibres. On the bone surface, collagen fibres are arranged in regular concentric lamellae which produces birefringence. Collagen fibres are arranged randomly in newly made osteoid. Collagen interacts with other tissue components such as proteoglycans, glycoproteins and mineral. These are important in determining the characteristics of the tissue. Type I collagen

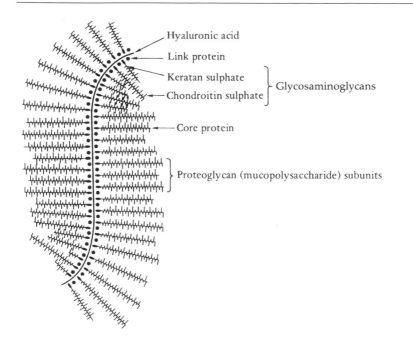

Figure 1.10 A diagram of a proteoglycan aggregate.

is found in other parts of the body but it is only in bone that it is mineralized.

Degradation of collagen within bone involves both collagenase activity and the removal of the mineral. Hydroxyapatite needs to be removed first since it protects collagen from denaturation. Bone collagen is broken down by a collagenase which cleaves the native triple helical molecule, then other proteases can further degrade the matrix. The resulting peptides and amino acids pass into the bloodstream and are excreted in the urine. These include hydroxyproline and hydroxylysine; their rate of excretion reflects the rate of collagen turnover. Since this is mainly of bone origin, it is also a measure of bone turnover.

Proteoglycans

These are complex macromolecules that permeate the ground substance of connective tissue throughout the body (see Figure 1.10). Proteoglycans contain acidic polysaccharide side-chains (glycosaminoglycans) attached to a central core protein. In bone, two types of glycosaminoglycan are found, predominantly chondroitin sulphate, but also heparan sulphate. The majority of glycosaminoglycans of bone are attached to the two small core proteins called PG-I (biglycan) and PG-II (decorin). PG-II binds to collagen fibrils and has a role in the regulation of collagen fibrillogenesis. The exact function of these small proteoglycans is not clear but they are probably important for the integrity of most connective tissue matrixes.

A large proteoglycan, aggrecan, is predominantly in articular cartilage. It is composed of a core protein with a large number of glycosaminoglycan side-chains and covalently attached oligosaccharides. The glycosaminoglycan chains, which comprise approximately 90% of the total mass of the macromolecule, are keratan sulphate and chondroitin sulphate. These proteoglycan macromolecules form aggregates when they are secreted into the extracellular matrix. The aggregates are formed by an interaction between a long-chain polysaccharide, hyaluronic acid, which consist of repeat units of *N*-acetylglucosamine and glucuronic acid; aggrecan; and α-link protein and create a highly hydrated network between collagen fibres. They have an overall negative charge, consequently binding large numbers of cations. This large polyelectrolyte structure, surrounded by small cations, determines the properties of a proteoglycan and its resistance to permeability by other ions.

Glycoproteins

These differ from proteoglycans in the nature of their carbohydrate side-chains, which do not contain regularly repeating disaccharide chains. They usually consist of relatively small numbers of monosaccharide residues, but have a wide variety of sugars. The side-chains may be short and straight with only two or three residues in each or they can be larger branching structures. In bone, the most relevant glycoproteins are alkaline phosphatase, osteonectin and the cell attachment proteins which include sialoproteins.

Osteocalcin (previously called bone-Gla protein)

Osteocalcin is predominantly confined to bone and accounts for up to 20% of the noncollagenous proteins in adult bone. It is synthesized by osteoblasts. It is also found in platelets and megakaryocytes. The serum osteocalcin level can be used as a marker of bone turnover and osteoblastic activity.[1] The structure of this 6000 dalton protein has been determined. The small molecule contains two stretches of α-helix and two regions of β-pleated sheet. It contains three residues of glutamic acid that are γ-carboxylated by a vitamin K-dependent mechanism. Osteocalcin has a high affinity for hydroxyapatite. It has a role in regulating bone growth and its serum level is a marker for osteoclast function.

Osteonectin

Osteonectin is an acidic glycoprotein and can compose up to 15% of the noncollagenous protein in bone.[2] It may be involved in the binding of bone mineral to collagenous matrix.

Bone morphogenetic proteins (BMP)

Bone morphogenetic proteins, originally investigated by Urist and colleagues,[3] are a family of proteins belonging to the transforming growth factor-β superfamily. They can be extracted from bone, dentine, osteosarcomata or metastases of prostate cancer. More than nine have been identified.

There are many other proteins which are found in bone and which may have regulatory effects.

Bone mineral and mineralization

Mature bone mineral is hydroxyapatite. Type I collagen by itself does not initiate mineralization. Mineralization of osteoid bone matrix clearly depends on other factors, such as the spatial arrangement of the collagen molecules or, more likely, the contribution of matrix noncollagenous substances such as phosphoproteins and sialoproteins. High energy phosphate bonds are thought to transfer to the collagen fibrils in an orderly fashion depending on the initiating proteins, possibly at free side-chains containing lysine or hydroxylysine. Newly precipitated free calcium phosphate is amorphous and it seems likely that the formation and crystallization of calcium hydroxyapatite around the collagen fibres of bone is determined by the shielding proteins. Concentrations of calcium and phosphate ions in extracellular fluid are adequate to induce crystallization and it is a paradox that other tissues do not normally calcify. Inhibitors to calcification, such as certain proteoglycans, carbonate, citrate and pyrophosphate, must be important in maintaining calcium solubility. These inhibitors must in some way be removed or disabled to allow calcification to occur. One occasional feature of osteoporosis is that the aorta may be heavily calcified while the spine loses calcium. Osteoblastic alkaline phosphatase may be important in enzymatically removing nonstructural pyrophosphate to allow mineralization.

Hydroxyapatite crystals lie within the holes in the collagen fibrils and, as crystal growth occurs, the mineralization spreads, resulting in the formation of mature, fully calcified bone. Following formation of osteoid there is a lag of 10 to 15 days, after which mineralization begins and rapidly reaches two-thirds. Ossification of the final third of the osteoid may take several months to complete.

Calcium which is taking part in the earliest stages of bone mineralization binds strongly to tetracycline. This is subsequently incorporated into the calcification front and can readily be detected by fluorescence microscopy which is used to assess bone formation (see Fig. 3.15).

The second commonest cation in bone mineral is magnesium and there are also small amounts of sodium.

Traces of fluoride are essential. Animals reared on a totally fluorine-free diet cannot make proper bone. Bone mineral chemistry is such that many divalent heavy metal ions taken into the body are deposited in bone in trace amounts. These include strontium, lead and radium. The removal of lead from the blood into the skeleton is an important scavenging mechanism in chronic lead poisoning.

Calcium

The total body calcium is about 1300 g, 99.9% of which is in the bones. Calcium is also bound to proteins, particularly plasma albumin. Calcium ions are essential for the proper function of all living cells (see Table 1.2), and

Table 1.2   Physiological processes involving calcium

1	*Bone formation*	Structural component Calcium pool
2	*Metabolism*	Cell activation Membrane transport Enzyme function Response to hormones Renal tubular function
3	*Glandular function*	Exocrine secretion
4	*Nerve conduction*	Central Peripheral
5	*Muscular contraction*	Voluntary muscle Smooth muscle Cardiac muscle
6	*Haemostatic control*	Platelet function Cofactor in clotting cascade
7	*Skin integrity*	

the concentration of ionized calcium in the blood is precisely regulated by feedback mechanisms acting through the parathyroid glands. Calcium in the blood and in the rest of the body fluids amounts to about 25 mmol (1 g), and is in dynamic equilibrium with protein-bound calcium and the surface layers of calcium fixed in the skeleton as hydroxyapatite. The chief sources of calcium in the diet are milk and cheese, together with vegetables and greens when these are eaten in quantity, as well as water in hard-water districts. Only a proportion of dietary calcium is absorbed; but only a proportion of faecal calcium is unabsorbed, with the rest coming from calcium in the intestinal secretions into the gut lumen and passed on into the colon. In adults, up to 25 mmol (1 g) of calcium can be lost in the faeces every day and about half as much in the urine, depending on the composition of the diet (see Figure 1.11).

The calcium content of a food cannot be taken out of context with the other components

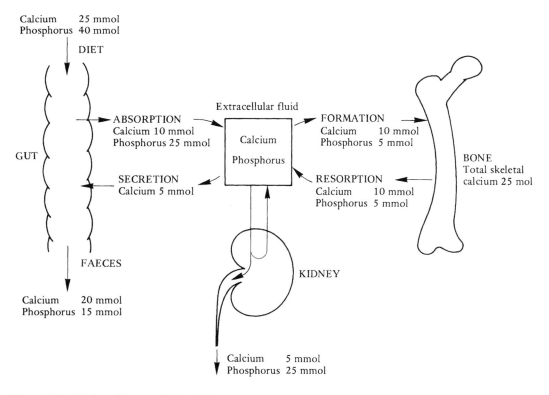

Figure 1.11   Daily calcium and phosphate turnover.

of the food (Table 1.3).[4] Calcium absorption is reduced by oxalates in leaf vegetables and by phytates in wholemeal flours. Calcium secretion into the urine is increased by sodium in the diet and reduced by potassium. It is also increased by aciduric flesh proteins.

Phosphorus

The second most common element of bone is phosphorus, which is similarly, although to a lesser extent, in equilibrium with body phosphate elsewhere. Dietary phosphate is ubiquitous and between 50 and 80% appears in the urine to a total of 14–48 mmol (1–1.5 g) of inorganic phosphate per 24 hours in adults.

Some phosphorus in the urine is derived from organic phosphates. The rate of filtration of phosphate from the blood into the urine is under the control of PTH. Increased PTH activity causes increased urinary loss of phosphate which in turn is compensated for by increased resorption of calcium and phosphate from the bones. In consequence, parathyroid overactivity is characterized by increases in urinary phosphate clearance and in the level of serum calcium. Aluminium hydroxide antacids bind phosphate in the gut and reduce absorption, eventually leading to increased mobilization of calcium and phosphate from bones. Phosphate and calcium are excreted in approximately equimolar

Table 1.3   Sources of dietary calcium, mg/100 g and bioavailability

	Ca	K	Na
Fruit	7–20	100–400	1–12
Vegetables – leaf[a,b]	50–150	200–500	4–150
– root[b]	25–50	300–400	3–50
Nuts[b]	50–200	400–900	3–30
Bread –fortified white	84	105	507
– unfortified white	43	90	580
– wholemeal[c]	84	256	530
Milk – whole	133	139	75
– dried skimmed	1300	150	53
Cheese (Cheddar)[d,e]	750	82	700
Soya flour, medium fat[b]	244	2025	—
Meats and poultry[e]	5–10	100–400	65
Fish[e]	5–60	100–400	100

Bioavailability: [a] reduced by oxalates, especially in spinach; [b]increased by potassium content; [c]reduced by 50% by phytates; [d]decreased by high salt content; [e]decreased by sulphur amino acid metabolites.

amounts in the faeces, but four to five times as much phosphate as calcium is excreted in the urine (see Figure 1.11).

Hydroxyapatite

The chemical composition of hydroxyapatite is $Ca_{10}(PO_4)_6(OH)_2$. The microcrystals of hydroxyapatite can be appreciated as such only under electron microscopy. Under light microscopy they appear amorphous. In bone they are arranged in a regular fashion corresponding to the periodicity of the linear collagen molecules to which they are bound. Osteoblasts secrete procollagen fibrils which assemble themselves extracellularly into collagen fibres. In the micro-environment of the bone surface (which is possibly supersaturated for calcium ions and phosphate) crystal nucleation begins immediately in regular arrays along the fibre. Microscopically similar crystals, not bound to collagen, are found in other areas of calcification in the body, for example, in the walls of blood vessels or in the supraspinatus tendon. In osteoarthritis, similar crystals are occasionally found free in the synovial fluid.

BONE GROWTH, MODELLING, REMODELLING AND REPAIR

Bone growth

The framework of the skeleton is apparent early in fetal development, long before mineralization. The long bones attain their future shape and proportions and left–right symmetry by about 26 weeks of gestation.

The skeleton of a new-born baby has about 25 g of calcium, acquired from the maternal placental circulation. If this were acquired at an even rate throughout gestation, the demand could be met from the diet, but demand increases to about 200 mg per day towards the end of pregnancy and there is a measurable loss of maternal bone density, which is normally quickly restored after the birth.

Bones grow in size during the first two decades of life, with a spurt during adolescence. This is followed by a period of consolidation. Peak adult bone mass is reached at about the age of 35 years for cortical bone and a little earlier for trabecular bone. The long bones grow in length at their epiphyses, the growth plates, but they also increase in diameter by endosteal resorption and periosteal apposition.

The size and shape of each bone and of the whole skeleton are genetically predetermined but the expression of this potential is influenced by growth and the environment. Endocrine factors, nutrition, physical forces and local growth factors all contribute. The modelling of growth results in the macroarchitectural features of the skeleton and allows it to adjust to the mechanical demands placed upon it. It is at this stage of growth that abnormalities of motor function, such as poliomyelitis and cerebral palsy result in the greatest abnormalities of skeletal shape.

There is wide variation in skeletal size both within and between races. Genetic factors are important but difficult to separate from environmental influences such as dietary habits and physical activity. Black people have larger, denser bones than whites, while Chinese have a small skeletal mass. However, correction of their low calcium diet has increased the average height of the Japanese and in Serbia a higher dietary intake of calcium has been shown to be associated with a higher bone mass (see page 214).[5]

Remodelling

In the adult there is a continuous turnover of bone, which enables it to repair any trabecular microdamage that occurs and to adjust its strength according to the mechanical stresses to which it is subjected. There is a linked cycle of bone resorption followed by bone formation. Whatever an agent does to bone resorption, in time there is a tendency for it to do the same to formation, so there is as yet no single factor which indefinitely continues to cause accumulation or loss of bone mineral. This coupling of formation and resorption can be observed on histological examination to occur in discrete packets. Remodelling of compact

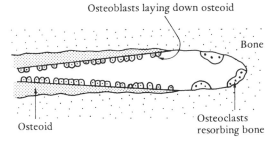

Figure 1.12   A diagram of a cutting cone with osteoclasts resorbing bone followed by osteoblasts depositing new osteoid, which subsequently becomes calcified.

bone is first done by osteoclasts which, within about eight days, form a cutting cone and move progressively through older mineralized bone to create a cavity for a new Haversian system (see Figure 1.12). Distal to this cutting cone, the newly excavated canal is colonized by a vascular stroma and poorly differentiated cells. Further back there are active plump osteoblasts depositing new lamellae. Successive cycles of resorption and formation result in the multiple lamellae of the Haversian system. In trabecular bone, osteoclastic resorption forms Howship's lacunae which are then filled by active osteoblasts that replace the bone. The cavity formed by the osteoclasts may take up to two months to remineralize. There is a much faster rate of bone turnover in trabecular bone than in cortical bone.

These coupled functional units of osteoclasts and osteoblasts have been called bone multicellular units (BMUs). They are asynchronous, so resorption at one site is balanced by formation at another, with no net weakening of the skeleton.

The local coupling between resorption and formation keeps an overall constant bone mass in the adult on a week-to-week basis. Over the course of the months or years, however, general or local influences can override this local coupling, and a low bone mass (i.e., osteoporosis) will arise if resorption exceeds formation.[6] Turnover rate will influence how rapidly this loss will occur. In the osteoporosis that follows oophorectomy there is a rapid turnover rate caused partly by increase in the rate of bone resorption by individual BMUs but principally by an increase in the number of actively remodelling BMUs. This means that a greater proportion of the bone will be occupied by BMUs with an increase in young bone which is only weakly mineralized. Resorption in cortical bone results in more and wider Haversian canals with increased cortical porosity, and in trabecular bone there is a perforation of trabecular plates and loss of connectivity of the trabeculae with an increased number of spicules.

Rates of bone turnover

The loss of bone mass which leads to osteoporosis is the result of the daily rate of bone resorption exceeding, perhaps by only a minute amount, the rate of bone formation. Within this relationship of formation and resorption or bone turnover lie the extremes of high turnover and low turnover. High turnover osteoporosis is exemplified in women who have undergone oophorectomy. Low turnover occurs in men and women over 75 years old. The typical outcome in high turnover osteoporosis is collapse fracture(s) of the spine. In contrast, the typical expression of low turnover osteoporosis is fracture of the femoral neck.

Many factors affect the modelling and remodelling of bone: age, disease, diet, hormones and mechanical stress[7] (Table 1.4).

Wolff stated in 1899 that bones form and remodel in response to the forces applied to them.[8] The orientation of trabeculae changes according to the stress. The thickness of cortex can change by variation in the rates of endosteal absorption and periosteal formation.

Immobilization of the whole body by bed-rest, or by weightlessness in space flight,

Table 1.4   Bone turnover in osteoporosis

Type of osteoporosis	High turnover	Low turnover
Oestrogen deficiency	+	
Postoophorectomy		
Postmenopausal under 65		
Anorexia		
Young female over-exercise syndrome		
Hyperprolactinaemia		
Idiopathic in young women	+	
Idiopathic in young men	+	
Juvenile idiopathic osteoporosis	+	
Pregnancy associated	+	
Glucocorticoid excess and Cushing's syndrome	+	
Thyrotoxicosis and thyroxine excess	+	
Over 75, men		+
Over 75, women		+

causes a rapid general loss of bone mass. Immobilization of a limb by splinting, paralysis or pain will have a local effect. In contrast, repeated exercise results in increased bone mass and strength, particularly of the most stressed bones; thus elite female athlete runners have significantly greater bone mass in their legs compared with rowers and dancers.[9] Experimental removal of the ulna in a sheep results in the rapid compensatory hypertrophy of the radius as it responds to the increased stress.[10]

Repair of fractures

Microscopically visible trabecular fractures with associated microcallus are continually occurring in bone and being repaired. This damage increases with age.

When the bone itself is fractured the fracture site fills with blood clot followed by granulation tissue containing capillaries, fibroblasts and progenitor cells. These progenitor cells proliferate and differentiate to form osteoblasts, which synthesize a matrix of woven bone and initiate its mineralization. This forms the callus and restores function. Callus becomes replaced over the next two to four years by lamellar bone continuous with the adjacent pre-existing lamella bone. Remodelling then occurs and the original shape of the bone is restored, rapidly in children but more slowly in later life. Repair of a fracture of osteoporotic bone occurs at a normal rate, but repair in osteomalacia results in poorly mineralized callus and in osteogenesis imperfecta there is abnormal remodelling.

CONTROL OF BONE GROWTH, COMPOSITION AND MASS

The normal growth and remodelling of the skeleton are dependent on systemic and local growth factors, on the supply of raw materials, and on the mechanical loading of the skeleton.[7,11–13]

There are many stages and ways in which the formation of a bone can be affected (Tables 1.5–1.8). First is the condensation of primitive mesenchymal cells that become the bone. The next stage is the proliferation and differentiation of chondrocytes which precedes the mineralization of matrix, and finally the differentiation of the osteoblasts and osteoclasts. This sequence of events must be under the control of morphogenetic and paracrine substances.

Once bone is formed it grows by remodelling and there must be systemic factors which co-ordinate periosteal formation and endosteal resorption. The symmetrical fusion of epiphyses in both sides of the skeleton must be co-ordinated by systemic factors for balanced growth to occur. Bone responds in density and strength to local stresses and this too must be under local control, but systemic factors are

Table 1.5   Levels of control of bone growth, composition and mass

1	*Molecular*, by collagen genes
2	*Cellular*, by osteoblastic and osteoclastic proliferation, differentiation and activity
3	*Tissue*, by coupling between osteoblastic and osteoclastic activity
4	*Organ*, by response to hormones and to loading

Table 1.6   Possible mechanism of control of bone composition

Formation

| Osteoblastic activity | Activation of resting cells
Proliferation and differentiation of preosteoblasts
Rate of matrix formation
Duration of matrix formation
Regulation of mineralization |
| *Mineralization* | Nucleation
Calcium and phosphate levels and factors controlling these |

Resorption

| Osteoclastic activity | Activation
Rate of resorption
Duration of resorption
Coupling with osteoblastic activity |

Table 1.7   Factors regulating bone formation and resorption

Calcium-regulating hormones
Parathyroid hormone
1,25-Dihydroxy-vitamin D_3
Calcitonin

Systemic hormones
Glucocorticoids
Growth hormone
Somatomedins
Thyroxine
Sex hormones

Cytokines and local growth factors (see Table 1.8)

Table 1.8   Effects of osteotropic cytokines on bone

Cytokine	Abbreviation	In vitro	In vivo
Interleukin-1	IL-1	Resorption	Resorption, hypercalcaemia
Tumour necrosis factor	TNF	Resorption	Resorption, hypercalcaemia
Leukotrienes	LT	Resorption	Resorption, hypercalcaemia
Interleukin-6	IL-6	Minimal resorption	Mild hypercalcaemia
Leukaemia inhibitory factor	LIF	Resorption	?
Transforming growth factor-β	TGF-β	Resorption ↓,↑	Formation
Interleukin-1 receptor antagonist	IL-1 ra	Resorption ↓	Resorption ↓, hypercalcaemia ↓
Monocyte-macrophage colony stimulating factor	M-CSF	Osteoclast formation	Osteoclast formation
Transforming growth factor-α	TGF-α	Resorption	Osteoclast progenitor cell replication
Bone morphogenetic protein	BMP	Osteoblast differentiation	Formation

Adapted from Mundy.[17]
↓, decrease; ↑, increase.

able to override the local balance, as for example when oestrogen deficiency leads to a generalized loss of bone mass (see Figure 1.13).

These control mechanisms, acting systemically or locally, have been intensively studied at molecular, cellular, tissue and organ levels, but there is as yet only limited knowledge about the control of bone growth and morphogenesis. Remote control of subperiosteal new growth is dramatically illustrated in pulmonary hypertrophic osteoarthropathy. In the presence of chronic pulmonary disease, a painful reflex hyperaemia develops in peripheral bones followed by formation of new subperiosteal woven bone. The afferent arm of the reflex is the vagus nerve and ipsilateral vagotomy reduces the periosteal blood flow within minutes. The efferent arm is humoral, but by what substance(s) is unknown.

At a molecular level, cDNA probes to several of the collagen genes permit the study of factors that affect collagen synthesis. Some hormonal control is exerted at the level of transcription of mRNA from the collagen genes. Abnormalities of the synthesis or composition of collagen have been found in

diseases of bone such as osteogenesis imperfecta by these techniques.

Pure populations of normal osteoblasts and osteoclasts can be immortalized by transfection with viral oncogenes so that they do not lose their phenotype on prolonged culture and are thus available for the study of the effect of humoral agents at cellular level. Most work over the last 25 years has been with tissue cultures. These have the disadvantage in that it is difficult to identify the cells that are responding. Cultures of rodent fetal or juvenile calvaria or limb bones have also been used, but the results are not necessarily applicable to human tissue. In rodents, unlike in man, skeletal growth decelerates with age but never stops.

Techniques used to study bone formation and resorption include histology, histochemistry, electron microscopy, enzymology, biochemistry and time lapse cinematography. Histomorphometry has permitted the study of the BMUs, which some consider to be the most relevant functional unit of bone turnover.

Changes in mass of the skeleton as a whole or in part can be measured in vivo, and

Table 1.9 The effects of calcitonin, PTH and vitamin D (and metabolites) on mineral metabolism*

Effect	Calcitonin	PTH	Vitamin D
Intestinal			
Calcium absorption	↓?	↑	↑
Phosphate absorption	?	?	↑
Renal			
Phosphate excretion	↑	↑	↓
Calcium excretion	↑	↓	↓
Skeletal			
Calcium mobilization	↓	↑	↑
Mineralization of bone matrix			↑
Others			
Plasma levels of calcium	↓	↑	↑
Plasma levels of phosphate	↓	↓	
Body weight	?	?	↑

*After Urist MR ed. *Fundamental and clinical bone physiology*. (JB Lippincott: Philadelphia (1980).

turnover can be estimated by biochemical indices or by bone biopsy (see Chapter 3).

Ions

Calcium and phosphate ions are required for normal bone formation. Several hormones maintain their serum concentrations. Phosphate deficiency and perhaps calcium deficiency can impair mineralization. Calcium deficiency may also result in increased resorption, bone being used as a reservoir from which to maintain extracellular and intracellular calcium concentrations. Phosphate may act as a regulator of bone metabolism. In vitro it stimulates mineralization and matrix formation.

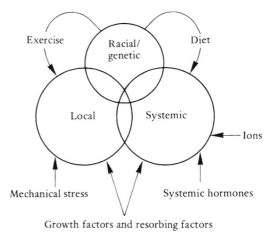

Figure 1.13 Factors influencing bone growth, composition and mass.

Calcium-regulating hormones

The physiological effects of the calcium-regulating hormones calcitonin, parathyroid hormone (PTH) and vitamin D metabolites in relation to mineral metabolism are shown in Table 1.9.

Parathyroid hormone

Parathyroid hormone is a hormone synthesized by the chief cells of the parathyroid gland. The short half-life 34-amino terminal fragment is the biologically active part of this 84-amino acid polypeptide hormone. Physiologically, PTH is the most important regulator of extracellular calcium concentration and a fall in serum calcium results in its increased secretion. This maintains the serum calcium by actions on bone, intestine and kidney (Table 1.9). Some of its effects on bone are therefore indirect. The way in which the cells of the parathyroid glands respond to decreased plasma levels of calcium is not known.

PTH stimulates osteoclasts to resorb bone, with an increase in their numbers and activities shown by a rapid increase in their ruffled borders. This is mediated by other bone cells, most probably osteoblasts, since isolated osteoclasts do not respond and they contain no PTH receptors. A direct effect of PTH on osteoblasts has been demonstrated in cell and organ culture. When isolated osteoblasts are treated with PTH they secrete factor(s) that stimulate osteoclasts to resorb bone. In spite of these demonstrated activities, PTH administration in vivo can be accompanied by some bone deposition. Indeed the N-terminal 1-34 peptide of parathormone (but not the parent hormone) is the only substance known to be able to promote the regrowth of normal-looking trabecular bone where this has been removed by the osteoporotic process.

Parathyroid hormone has several actions on the kidney. It increases calcium resorption mainly in the distal tubule and decreases phosphate resorption in the proximal tubule. This increases serum calcium but prevents an increase in the calcium phosphate product and with it the redeposition of calcium in bone mineral. A third effect of PTH on the kidney is to increase 1,25-dihydroxy-vitamin D_3 synthesis by the proximal convoluted tubule with a subsequent increase in intestinal calcium absorption. PTH has no direct effect on the gut.

Vitamin D (Fig. 1.14)

In the 1920s an antirachitic factor was identified in cod liver oil and called vitamin D. It was soon found that the antirachitic activity of this vitamin could be induced by UV radiation of affected animals or of their food, in particular the sterol fraction. The structure of vitamin D was then identified and rickets, which had been a major medical problem, was virtually eradicated. Over the last 15 years a large number of metabolites of vitamin D have been identified. 1,25-dihydroxy-vitamin D_3 appears to carry out all the functions of the vitamin D hormone system.[14]

The natural form of vitamin D is cholecalciferol, which is designated vitamin D_3. It is present in fish oils and dairy products, and is formed in the skin by the action of UV light on 7-dehydrocholesterol. The synthetic form of vitamin D is ergocalciferol, derived from the irradiation of a plant sterol. It is designated vitamin D_2. Vitamins D_2 and D_3 are equally active in humans.

Vitamins D_2 and D_3 are hydroxylated by the liver to the 25-hydroxy metabolites, the major circulating forms, but these cannot stimulate intestinal calcium transport or bone calcium mobilization. In the 1970s, the 1,25-dihydroxy metabolite (calcitriol), the most potent, was identified. It is formed in the renal mitochondria by the enzyme 1-α-hydroxylase. This enzyme is found only in the kidney, and this organ is therefore an important site of regulation of vitamin D activity. The other metabolite that is important is 24,25-dihydroxy-vitamin D_3 which is produced by the kidney and has physiological effects different from 1,25-dihydroxy-vitamin D_3.

The metabolites 25-hydroxy-vitamin D and 1,25-dihydroxy-vitamin D_3 circulate largely bound to a carrier protein. 1,25-dihydroxy-vitamin D_3 is rapidly cleared from the blood to accumulate in the target tissues. It acts on the intestine and on the skeleton to maintain the blood calcium supply, but receptors are found on cells from a wide variety of tissues, including the immune system, implying a wider

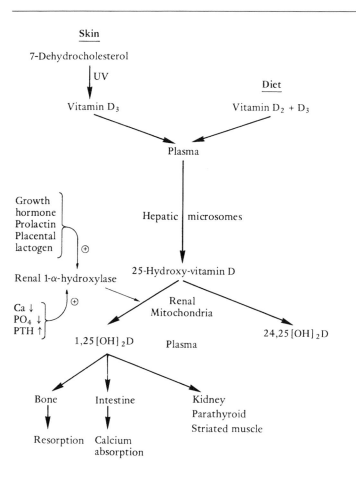

Figure 1.14   Vitamin D metabolism.

physiological role and vitamin D congeners are used in psoriasis and myeloproliferative disorders. It is the gut, however, that is the principal site of 1,25-dihydroxy-vitamin D_3 activity, increasing calcium and phosphate absorption. It also has direct and indirect effects on bone, often in conjunction with PTH. Osteoblasts express the vitamin D receptor and 1,25-dihydroxy-vitamin D_3 modulates cellular proliferation and differentiation and inhibits Type I collagen synthesis. 1,25-dihydroxy-vitamin D_3 stimulates bone resorption probably by direct stimulation of precursor cells to differentiate into mature

osteoclasts. Vitamin D deficiency impairs mineralization of bone matrix, leading to widened uncalcified osteoid in adults which is corrected by replenishment. The mechanism of this process is unclear but may be mainly due to actions on the intestine and the absorption of calcium and phosphate. Renal 1-α-hydroxylase activity regulates 1,25-dihydroxy-vitamin D_3 production. It is altered by factors that are involved in the regulation of plasma calcium (PTH, plasma calcium and phosphate), in increasing 1,25-dihydroxy-vitamin D_3 production during growth, pregnancy and lactation (growth hormone, prolactin and insulin) and, finally, in maintaining vitamin D activity despite variable exposure to sunlight.

Since vitamin D is important for normal bone growth, its direct inhibition of osteoblastic collagen synthesis and its stimulation of bone resorption appear contradictory. It is possible that in vivo bone resorption is increased by 1,25-dihydroxy-vitamin D_3 only when dietary calcium deficiency is too severe to be compensated for by the improved efficiency of calcium absorption following the increase in 1,25-dihydroxy-vitamin D_3 synthesis.

Inadequate calcium absorption will also lead to increased PTH secretion in vivo, and to increased bone resorption. Few diets contain the recommended daily allowance of vitamin D, 90% of which is normally made in the skin by the action of sunlight. Consequently, vitamin D blood levels are markedly seasonal but summer excess can be stored in fat and liver cells for the winter.

Calcitonin

This 32-amino acid polypeptide hormone is produced by the C cells of the thyroid gland which originate from the neural crest. Its existence was first postulated in 1962 by Copp. The hormone and the gene have been sequenced, and the hormone synthesized by recombinant DNA technology.

Calcitonin is cleaved from a large precursor polyprotein within which it is flanked by a 21-amino acid peptide, katacalcin, which also has a potent calcium-lowering effect.[15] Its secretion is regulated by the plasma calcium level. A high serum calcium increases calcitonin secretion, and a low serum calcium reduces it. Secretion is also stimulated by 1,25-dihydroxy-vitamin D_3.

Genes for calcitonins have been strongly conserved in vertebrate evolution. Salmon calcitonin, which is active in man, is thought to be important in the regulation of the biochemical *milieu intérieur* when the fish swim from the salt water of the oceans to the fresh water of the streams for spawning. In man, the skeleton is the only proven physiologically important target. Calcitonin directly inhibits osteoclastic bone resorption and does not increase the deposition of calcium in the skeleton in vivo, unless bone turnover is high. It produces little change in serum calcium owing to the compensating response of the other calcium-regulating hormones. It does not normally have a sustained effect and this escape may be because of a down-regulation of the receptor.

The physiological role of calcitonin may be either to respond to short-lived changes in serum calcium consequent on dietary loading in order to prevent hypercalcaemia and hypercalcuria, or to protect the skeleton from the actions of PTH and vitamin D when calcium is required.

Calcitonin has a powerful inhibitory effect on osteoclasts, which have specific receptors, producing a decrease in their ruffled border and a rise in intracellular cyclic AMP. Seen under the microscope the effect of calcitonin on living osteoclasts is one of rapid shrinking—rather like the effect of putting salt on a slug! No direct effect has been found on other bone cells and the only other known action of calcitonin that may be of physiological importance is the enhancement of 1-α-hydroxylase enzyme activity in the renal proximal tubule with increased 1,25-dihydroxy-vitamin D_3 synthesis.

Glucocorticoids

Glucocorticoids have both direct and indirect effects on the skeleton. Their effects are concentration-dependent. Supraphysiological concentrations markedly inhibit pre-osteoblastic replication, impair skeletal growth, suppress osteoblastic bone formation, decrease intestinal calcium absorption and decrease bone mass, but physiological concentrations play a permissive role in normal osteoblastic function. Glucocorticoid receptors occur in bone cells.

Loss of bone mass is inevitable with the continued administration of more than 8 mg of prednisolone per day, and histological studies have shown decreased bone formation and increased bone resorption activity. In vivo, glucocorticoids administered in excess have a direct inhibitory effect on osteoblastic activity. They decrease collagen synthesis and suppress progenitor cell proliferation. Increased bone resorption might be expected to result from direct stimulation of osteoclasts but, in vitro, osteoclast activity is actually inhibited. An alternative explanation is that increased resorption is an indirect effect of glucocorticoids, mediated by the increase in PTH in response to the impairment of intestinal calcium absorption caused by glucocorticoids. This is supported by the observation that parathyroidectomy abolishes the osteoclast response to glucocorticoids in animals, but it is not known how they impair calcium absorption.

Growth hormone

Growth hormone stimulates growth of the skeleton and is probably mediated by the synthesis and secretion of somatomedins. Growth hormone and growth hormone releasing agent increase markers of osteoblastic activity but not bone density.[16]

Thyroid hormone

Excess of thyroid hormone leads to increased bone turnover, hypercalcaemia, decreased PTH, decreased 1,25-dihydroxy-vitamin D$_3$, decreased intestinal calcium absorption and, eventually, to osteoporosis. Increases in serum alkaline phosphatase, urinary hydroxyproline and deoxypyridinoline cross-links reflect the high bone turnover and increased bone resorption. The stimulation of resorption is the only major direct effect of thyroid hormone shown on bone. Thyroid hormone deficiency is associated with impaired skeletal turnover and

growth. Thyroid hormones also stimulate cartilage growth, both alone and synergistically with somatomedin.

Sex hormones

Sex hormones have marked effects on the skeleton and deficiencies are associated with low bone mass in both children and adults. This is most evident following loss of circulating oestrogens in surgically induced premature menopause (see page 187). Androgens are also important and are responsible for the pubertal growth spurt. Oestrogens act on the skeleton via the osteoblasts, which contain nuclear receptors, and oestradiol-17 reduces the production of bone-damaging cytokines (see Chapter 8).

Cytokines

Cytokines are locally active factors that are formed by immunologically competent cells. They have many activities including that on bone, and osteotropic cytokines are involved in both normal and abnormal bone modelling (Table 1.8).[17]

Interleukins-1α and 1β (IL-1α and β) are powerful stimulators of bone resorption. They affect osteoclasts at all stages of their lineage, for example by stimulating prostaglandin synthesis. The effects on osteoblasts are complex and may be implicated in bone loss and destruction in rheumatoid arthritis.

Tumour necrosis factor (TNF) and lymphotoxin (TNFβ) stimulate osteoclastic bone resorption, and stimulate cells at all stages of osteoclast lineage. TNF may cause hypercalcaemia in certain malignancies.

Transforming growth factor β (TGFβ) and the bone morphogenetic proteins (BMP) are all related molecules that have distinct effects on bone formation and resorption. TGFβ is released in its active form during bone resorption but its effects on formation are best known where it can stimulate osteoblast migration and proliferation of osteoblast precursors resulting in new bone formation. It has variously been shown to stimulate and inhibit bone resorption. Bone morphogenetic proteins have been extracted from bone matrix and are powerful stimulators of ectopic bone formation. They affect the differentiated function of osteoblasts.

Leukotrienes, the 5-lipoxygenase metabolites of arachadonic acid, stimulate osteoclastic bone resorption and leukotriene B4 acts both directly on isolated osteoclasts and also by causing fusion of osteoclast precursors. Their physiological role is not yet clear, but as they are produced in inflammatory tissues they may be responsible for related bone loss such as that associated with chronically infected gingiva.

Prostaglandins of the E-series stimulate bone resorption in organ cultures, and in vivo they may mediate bone resorption stimulated by systemic factors such as interleukin-1, TGFα and many others. Prostaglandins also have various effects on osteoblasts.

The effects of cytokines on bone and their role are clearly complicated and unresolved. There would appear to be redundancy of activities. They may act directly or indirectly and may mutually interact. Their role in coupling of formation and resorption and how they are controlled are clinically relevant questions.

Local growth factors

Epidermal (EGF), fibroblast (FGF) and platelet-derived (PDGF) growth factors have direct effects on bone and can be found in the circulation. They stimulate bone cell proliferation and PDGF increases protein synthesis. They also stimulate resorption by a prostaglandin-dependent mechanism, although EGF can independently stimulate resorption. Low concentrations of insulin-like growth factor (IGF) have been found in young men with osteoporosis and concentrations respond to IGF treatment.[18] Bone morphogenetic proteins (BMPs) are related to the transforming growth factor superfamily. They have been extracted from bone matrix and now more than nine have been identified.

CHANGES WITH AGE

Bone mass changes with age: both cortical and trabecular bone are lost. In cortical bone there is a widening of the Haversian canals on the endosteal surface with a failure to deposit new bone. This increases intracortical porosity. There is also a reduction in cortical thickness, especially in men. In trabecular bone there is a thinning of trabeculae with perforation and loss of connectivity with only spicules remaining. Thinned trabeculae may also sustain microfractures and the frequency with which these can be found postmortem increases with age. Impaired remodelling will slow their healing.

These changes are not uniform throughout the skeleton, however. This is best seen in the vertebrae where, with ageing, the horizontal trabeculae are lost first, followed later by the vertical trabeculae. There is also a rising incidence of fractures with age. Their relation to bone mass and factors influencing them are further discussed in Chapter 2.

PRACTICAL POINTS

- There is continuous turnover (remodelling) of bone in the adult, occurring in cycles of formation and resorption.

- Both high and low rates of turnover occur in osteoporosis.

- Osteoporosis (low bone mass) arises from an imbalance between formation and resorption.

- Many factors such as disease, diet, hormones and mechanical stress, affect bone remodelling.

- Immobilization causes rapid general loss of bone mass. Repeated exercise increases bone mass and strength, especially of the stressed bones.

- Mature bone mineral is hydroxyapatite. Its most important elements are calcium, phosphate and fluorine, all vital for healthy bone.

- The calcium-regulating hormones involved in bone are PTH, 1,25-dihydroxy-vitamin D_3 and calcitonin.

- Sex hormones have a significant effect on the skeleton and deficiencies are associated with low bone mass. Other hormones also have a role in bone maintenance.

- Other factors affecting bone growth and resorption include PGE_2, IL-1 and other cytokines.

REFERENCES

1. Price PA, Parthemore JG, Deftos LJ. New biochemical marker for bone metabolism. Measurement by radioimmunoassay of bone Gla protein in the plasma of normal subjects and patients with bone disease. *J Clin Invest* (1980), **66**: 878–83.

2. Termine JD, Kleinman HK, Whitson SW et al. Osteonectin, a bone-specific protein linking mineral to collagen. *Cell* (1981), **26**: 99–105.

3. Urist MR, Huo YK, Brownell AG et al. Purification of bovine bone morphogenetic protein by hydroxyapatite chromatography. *Proc Natl Acad Sci U S A* (1984), **81**: 271.

4. Lentner C ed. *Composition of foods: Geigy scientific tables*, eighth edition. CIBA-GEIGY: Basle (1981), **1**: 241–66

5. Matkovic V, Kostial K, Simonovic I et al. Bone status and fracture rates in two regions of Yugoslavia. *Am J Clin Nutr* (1979), **32**: 540–9.

6. Parfitt AM. The coupling of bone formation to bone resorption: a critical analysis of the concept and of its relevance to the pathogenesis of osteoporosis. *Metab Bone Dis Relat Res* (1984), **4**: 1–6.

7. Mundy GR. *Bone remodeling and its disorders*. Martin Dunitz: London (1995), p. 39.

8. Wolff J. Die Lehre von den functionellen Knochengestalt. *Virchows Arch* (1899), **156**: 256.

9. Wolman RL, Faulman L, Clark P et al. Different training patterns and bone mineral density of the femoral shaft in elite, female athletes. *Ann Rheum Dis* (1991), **50**: 487–9.

10. Lanyon LE, Rubin CT. Regulation of bone mass in response to physical activity. In: Dixon AS, Russell RRG, Stamp TCB eds. *Osteoporosis, a multi-disciplinary problem*. Roy Soc Med Int Congr & Symp Series, No. 55, Academic Press: London (1983), pp. 51–61.

11. Raisz L. Regulation of bone formation. *N Engl J Med* (1983), **309**: 29–35, 83–9.

12. Goldharber P. Degradation of bone. In: Panayi GS ed. *Scientific basis of rheumatology*. Churchill Livingstone: Edinburgh (1982), pp. 179–97.

13. Canalis E. The humoral and local regulation of bone formation. *Endocr Rev* (1983), **42**: 62–77.

14. Koshy KT. Vitamin D: an update. *J Pharm Sci* (1982), **71**: 137–53.

15. Hillyard C, Myers C, Abeyasekera G et al. Katacalcin: a new plasma calcium-lowering hormone. *Lancet* (1983), *ii*: 846–8.

16. Clemmesen B, Overgaard T, Riis B et al. Human growth hormone and human growth hormone releasing hormone: a double masked, placebo controlled study of their effects on bone metabolism in elderly women. *Osteoporos Int* (1993), **3**: 330–6.

17. Mundy GR, Boyce BF, Yoneda T et al. Cytokines and bone remodelling. In: Marcus R, Feldman D, Kelsey J eds. *Osteoporosis*. Academic Press: San Diego (1996), pp. 301–13.

18. Johansson AG, Lindh E, Ljunghall SJ. Insulin-like growth factor 1 stimulates bone turnover in osteoporosis. *Lancet* (1992), **339**: 1619.

RECOMMENDED READING

Marcus R, Feldman D, Kelsey J, Roodman GD eds. *Osteoporosis*. Academic Press: London (1996).

2 Osteoporosis: the concepts

EPIDEMIOLOGY

Epidemiology is the study of diseases in populations as opposed to individuals. It is concerned with prevalence of diseases, with their severity (in the sense of the disturbance caused to the community) and with the community response (in the sense of provision of resources for prevention and treatment). The epidemiology of osteoporosis poses special problems as it is not a disease that by itself causes complaint. People with osteoporosis do not seek medical aid until something happens—generally a fracture, less commonly loss of height or back pain. The loss of bone mass and architectural deterioration are silent. The level of recognition of osteoporosis, and hence estimates of its prevalence, depend upon the observer's standpoint, and each approach has its own usefulness within a certain context.

A public health physician who is concerned with preventing fractures and improving their management needs to know the number of people who have osteoporosis-related fractures, the *clinical prevalence*. His interest in the epidemiology of risk factors for reduced bone mass and strength is only in this context. The medical epidemiologist seeking to compare populations or communities for clues to aetiology will want to know the *biological prevalence*, the number of people who have a pathological degree of osteoporosis (as judged by appropriate age, sex and race-matched norms), whether or not the condition has led to clinical disease. A drug company, planning to market a treatment for osteoporosis will be mainly concerned with the *perceived prevalence*, that is the number of individuals in whom the diagnosis of osteoporosis is made, which is limited by awareness and availability of diagnostic tools.

Two other factors further complicate the task of assessing the prevalence of osteoporosis. Its clinical recognition generally requires a fracture, but this is an all-or-none phenomenon: either the subject has it or she does not. People sustain fractures for a variety of reasons, however. Slipping on icy pavements in winter is one, but this would hardly be relevant in comparing the burden of osteoporosis in northern and tropical countries. The second and probably more important factor is that at present the biological prevalence of osteoporosis can be measured only by methods that assess bone density, but this is a surrogate measure for bone strength and does not always bear a close and constant relationship to it. Access to this diagnostic tool is also limited in some populations.

This chapter will start by exploring the history and definition of osteoporosis and go on to discuss the different patterns of age-related fractures, the age-related changes in bone mass and the concepts of 'skeletal failure', 'fracture risk' and of 'peak bone mass'. It will be concerned with the relationship of bone strength to bone mass and with the types and contribution of trauma and 'unintentional injury'. Finally, it will look at the medical and social determinants of falls in the elderly and the cost to the community of osteoporosis itself and of measures designed to prevent it.

Definition and measurement

The terminology associated with osteoporosis was developed in the nineteenth century by German pathologists to distinguish osteomalacia, osteoporosis and osteitis fibrosa cystica. Later, when X-rays were available, osteoporosis was not readily distinguished from osteomalacia and the two were often considered together. In 1941, Fuller Albright[1] and colleagues defined osteoporosis pathologically as 'a condition in which there is lack of bone tissue, but that tissue which remains is fully calcified'. This differentiated it from osteomalacia, a condition involving failure of bone matrix mineralization, most frequently usually caused by deficiency in vitamin D or disturbance in its metabolism.

Definitions of osteoporosis and osteopenia that are now generally accepted, despite their limitations, and which have proved useful in practice are:

Clinical definition

Osteoporosis is a systemic skeletal disease characterized by low bone mass and micro-architectural deterioration of bone tissue, with a consequent increase in bone fragility and susceptibility to fracture.

Definitions useful for comparative purposes

The categories of the disease are defined in terms of bone mineral density and fractures:

- *Osteoporosis* is when the bone density measurement falls 2.5 or more standard deviations below the young adult mean for age and sex.
- *Severe or established osteoporosis* is the same but coupled with the presence of one or more fractures.
- *Osteopenia* (or low bone mass) is when the bone density lies between 1 and 2.5 standard deviations below the mean for young adults. It is sometimes used to describe a 'demineralized' X-ray, although this is a very unreliable way of determining reduced bone density.

Classification of osteoporosis

All osteoporosis should be considered secondary to some underlying condition until proved otherwise. The term 'primary osteoporosis' thus becomes a diagnosis by exclusion, while all chronic diseases which interfere with normal body physiology, whether of the heart, liver, kidneys, locomotor and nervous systems can be reflected in damage to the skeletal system. It is better to classify osteoporosis in terms of with or without identifiable causes (Table 2.1).

Skeletal failure

The concept of skeletal structural failure applies both to fractures of long bones and to compression fractures of trabecular bone. There are, however, different resource implications. Fractures of long bones are fractures with displacement; they imply medical, usually hospital, treatment and can be life-threatening. Compression fractures of the trabecular bone, exemplified by wedged or crushed fractures of vertebral bodies are fractures without displacement, are not life-threatening and seldom require treatment other than relief of pain. Long bone fractures

Table 2.1 Classification of osteoporosis

Osteoporosis without identifiable cause
- Idiopathic juvenile osteoporosis
- Osteoporosis in adults
  Idiopathic adult osteoporosis
  Senile osteoporosis

Osteoporosis with identifiable cause
- Osteoporosis associated with endocrine disease
  Hormone deficiency (e.g. hypogonadism, male and female, vitamin D deficiency)
  Hormone excess (e.g. glucocorticoid excess, hyperthyroidism, hyperprolactinaemia)
- Osteoporosis due to nutritional factors (commonly mixed forms of osteoporosis, osteomalacia and sometimes reactive hyperparathyroidism)
  Malabsorbtion syndromes
  Digestive abnormalities including chronic hepatic diseases
- Renal bone disease
- Osteoporosis due to immobilization, paralysis or disuse
- Osteoporosis due to inflammatory disorders (Crohn's disease, rheumatoid arthritis)
- Osteoporosis due to neoplastic disorders of bone marrow

The following conditions are associated with reduced bone density and should be considered in the differential diagnosis
- Hyperparathyroidism
- Osteomalacia
- Osteogenesis imperfecta

Adapted from Bröll, ref.2.

considerably outnumber clinically apparent compression fractures, yet in many medical minds the word osteoporosis is linked only to spinal compression fractures.

It becomes purely academic to discuss the definition of osteoporosis and its various risk factors, its development and means of prevention if both the public and medical practitioners do not recognize skeletal failure as a distinct phenomenon such as cardiac failure. All too frequently it is considered a 'natural' part of ageing when an old person breaks a hip following a minor fall in the house. There is a

need to increase awareness that most osteoporosis is an abnormal and potentially preventable phenomenon. Without this we will not progress with prevention.

To identify the risk factors for osteoporosis we need to look at large samples of the whole community. But are our measurement techniques good enough? Most of the techniques measure bone mass as this correlates with fragility. Some of these earlier techniques, however, measured bone mass in less relevant sites such as the metacarpus. Bone mass does correlate with fracture risk, particularly if measured at the future site of fracture, but the correlation is not sufficient to be predictive for the individual (Chapter 3). It is of demonstrable value in identifying risk factors in epidemiological studies. Alternatively, we can look at the structure of bone by biopsy but this procedure is restricted to the iliac crest, which is not the site of osteoporosis-related fractures and there is a large sampling error. Ultrasound techniques which are being developed and evaluated may give a measure of mass and structure as well as strength.

It we measure the clinical prevalence of osteoporosis we need to remember that the trauma responsible for the bone structural failure also varies. An old man with relatively strong bones may fracture falling off a stepladder while a bed-ridden woman with weak bones may fail to fracture if carefully nursed. Life is further complicated for the epidemiologist by the fact that some osteoporotic people will suffer more than one type of fracture during old age, and that many vertebral compression fractures do not come to notice if they are painless (only an X-ray survey would detect them).

In the assessment of a risk factor or of the merit of a treatment for osteoporosis, an effect on fracture rate must be demonstrated since this is the clearest manifestation of skeletal fragility. Fractures cause the socioeconomic burden of osteoporosis and local and central governmental agencies are increasingly aware of the financial savings to be made by reducing their incidence. But there is a problem. Any treatment for the prevention of osteoporosis must be shown to reduce fracture rates. But if, for example, women in a population have a lifetime risk of two in five of sustaining an osteoporosis-related fracture, then three in five of those women will not be at risk. For them preventative treatment is superfluous. This emphasizes the importance of identifying within the population those most at risk and reducing their vulnerability. Today, much osteoporosis research is directed at solving these problems.

AGE-RELATED FRACTURES

The age distribution of fractures is bimodal (see Figure 2.1).[3] After a peak in youth associated with trauma, the incidence per thousand falls, then rises in those over 50 years of age and continues to increase with age (see Figure 2.2).[4]

The site of fracture varies with age as does the type of precipitating trauma. In youth, fractures of long bones are common, usually following road traffic accidents or sporting injuries. With age, the incidence of fracture rises even though the precipitating trauma is less severe, often merely a fall from standing height. Younger men break their bones more often than young women, but older women fracture more often than older men.

The main age-related (and hence probably osteoporosis-related) fractures occur in the vertebral bodies, proximal femur, proximal humerus, distal forearm and pelvis (see Figures 2.2 and 2.3). The estimated lifetime risk in a 50-year-old, of hip, vertebral or distal forearm fracture is 13.1% in white men and 39.7% in white women. There is an increase in Colles' fracture of the wrist in women from the age of 45, about the time of the menopause, but no significant increase in men of the same age. Vertebral fractures become more frequent from the age of 50, particularly in women.

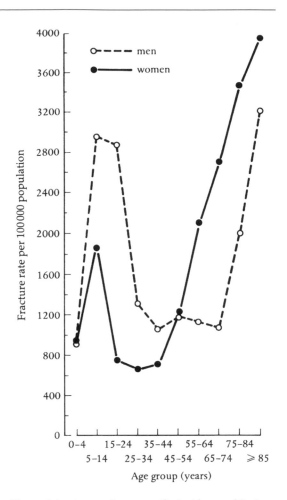

Figure 2.1   Age- and sex-specific incidence of limb fractures in Rochester, Minnesota, 1969–71.

Women have a lifetime risk of 15.6% of a vertebral fracture, but only one in three of these fractures will have presented clinically.[5] The comparable risk for men is 5.0%. One-fourth of white women 50 years and over have one or more vertebral fractures.[6] The incidence of fractures of the proximal femur increases rapidly in the elderly reaching rates of 3% per year among women aged 85 years and over,

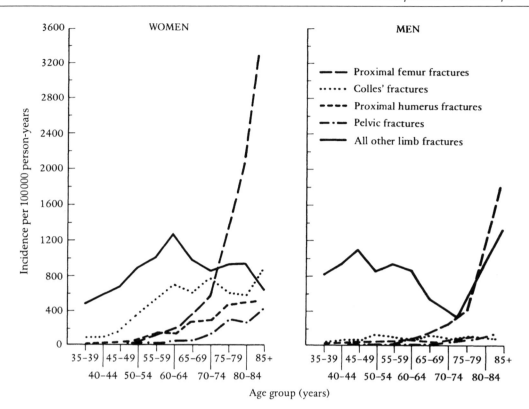

Figure 2.2 Age- and sex-specific incidence of various age-related fractures.

and 1.9% per year in men of a similar age. The rate is double in women than men at all ages, but because of the greater number of elderly women 80% of all hip fractures affect them. With increasing age, trochanteric fractures outnumber trans-cervical hip fractures in women. The reverse occurs in men. Worldwide there were an estimated 1.66 million hip fractures in 1990 and it is estimated that this will increase to 6.26 million by 2050.[7]

Colles', vertebral and hip fractures are interrelated in that patients who have sustained one have an increased risk of sustaining another at a different site, but the correlation between the various sites is less than one would expect if they were all a consequence of a generalized reduction in bone mass.

Medicosocial consequences

The consequences of this age-related increase in long bone fractures are enormous, both socioeconomically and regarding morbidity and mortality. Those who suffer them are often just managing to remain independent and self-sufficient, but a long bone fracture

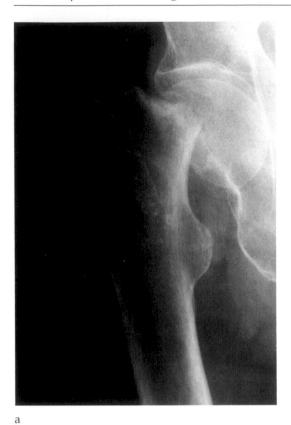
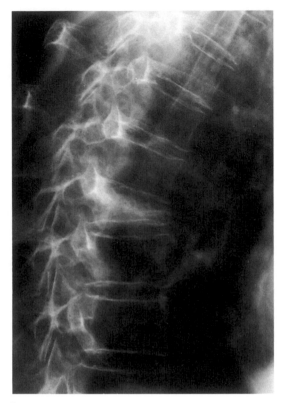

a

b

Figure 2.3   Various age-related fractures: (a) proximal femur; (b) vertebral wedge fracture; (c) distal radius; and (d) proximal humerus.

can put the full burden of care on to relatives and the rest of the community. In contrast, vertebral wedging and compression fractures lead to loss of height and occasionally to severe pain, but these fractures do not usually require much medical care or prolonged hospitalization. This does not mean that they are without morbidity and various measures of quality of life have been found to be adversely affected in those with vertebral fracture. Colles' fractures can cause considerable disability and temporary dependence on

others, but it is fractures of the neck of the femur which have the largest impact, requiring hospitalization and surgery, and many of those who fracture do not return to their previous environment. There is an overall reduction of survival in women of 10–20%, with the majority of excess deaths in the first six months. It is worse in men. Some of these deaths are due to complications of the fracture or to surgery. They may have lain on the floor unattended for a period following the fall, with the risk of developing a pressure sore or

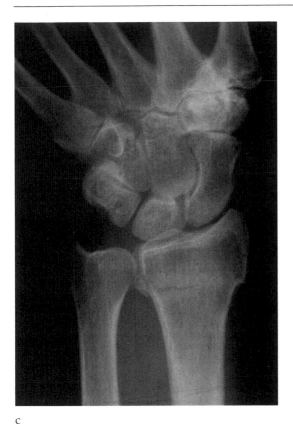

c

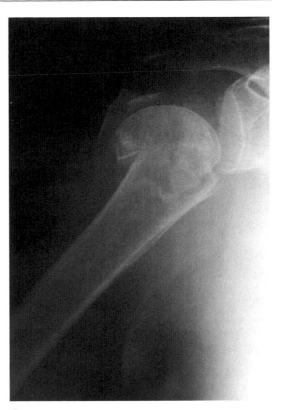

d

pneumonia. The subsequent immobilization in a hospital bed may lead to venous thrombosis and pulmonary embolism. Mortality is related to the length of time lying on the floor following a fall. A marked deterioration of mental state may follow such an episode. Deaths also relate to serious coexisting illnesses. Of those who survive, up to one-third are unable to return to their previous environment and need long-term care and support. Many have impaired mobility. Patients with fractures of the proximal femur occupy large numbers of expensive hospital and nursing home beds.

The cost to the community in human suffering and in money is considerable. The incidence of fracture of the neck of the femur has also been increasing in real terms, both in the UK and the USA, faster than the increase in the numbers of elderly people. There are some recent indications that the age-specific rate is now levelling off. Perhaps these changes reflect inadequate childhood nutrition of the cohort now elderly who grew up during the

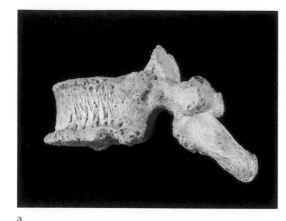

a

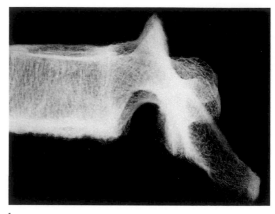

b

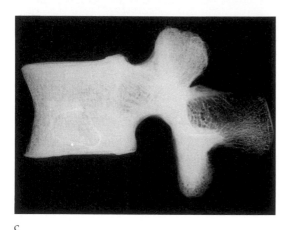

c

Figure 2.4 Vertebrae found in a Neolithic long barrow dated approximately 2500 BC. The osteoporotic vertebra (a and b) is compared to a normal vertebra (c) from the same excavation site.

First World War and the subsequent period of economic depression. This increase in fracture of the proximal femur in the growing population of the elderly means that the burden on the community will increase steadily unless effective means of preventing age-related fractures are found. The annual costs of osteoporosis are mainly those caused by hip fractures and these were estimated for England only £742 million (1992/3 prices),[8] and this did not include the costs of hip replacement.

Projections for future costs are daunting. Findings for other countries are similar.[9]

AGE-RELATED CHANGES IN BONE MASS

Following the growth of the skeleton, there is a period of consolidation over about 15 years, with further calcium accretion, decreased cortical porosity and increasing cortical thickening. Peak adult bone mass is attained at or before 35 years. Bone mass subsequently declines with ageing. This is a universal phenomenon, occurring in both sexes, in all races and in prehistory. Prehistoric adults lost bone whether they were hunters or farmers, or lived in sunny or cold climates. The skeletons from a Neolithic long barrow (see Figure 2.4) illustrate the characteristic loss of trabecular density of the vertebrae. In more recent times records giving the age at death together with skeletal material from a London Church, dating from 1729–1852, gave Lees and colleagues[10] the opportunity to compare bone loss with that of present day women. Today's women had less bone mass at the proximal femur than did the women of two centuries ago, both before and after the menopause. The differences were attributed to the much greater amount of physical activity in past times.

At all ages women have less mass per unit volume of bone than men. Premenopausally they have about 15% less compact bone corrected for bone size. With ageing this difference becomes more pronounced (see Figure 2.5).

Although we all lose bone with ageing, this loss is more rapid in postmenopausal women. The differential rate of bone loss from the various parts of the skeleton, its time of onset and the difference between men and women have not been fully ascertained, however, because of the limitations of methods of measurement available over the last 40 years (see Chapter 3). Over the last 10 years, dual energy densitometry and quantitative CT have been developed which allow measurement at a variety of clinically relevant sites and which separate cortical and trabecular changes. Longitudinal data are becoming available. Most sites that are measured comprise both cortical and trabecular bone: although one type of bone often predominates, the changes that are measured may not reflect solely the predominant component. Differential changes in cortical compared with trabecular bone and in the axial skeleton compared with the appendicular skeleton occur with ageing and with

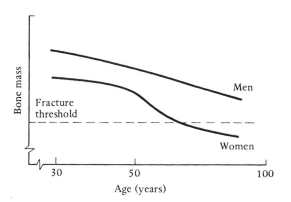

Figure 2.5 Women have a lower bone mass than men at all ages, with a period of rapid loss at the expected age of menopause. With age it is suggested that a threshold is crossed, with an increased risk of fracture.

treatment. Methods that have been used have looked at the whole skeleton by estimating the total body calcium or at isolated sites such as the cortex of the metacarpal bones, the trabecular bone volume at the iliac crest or the bone density at the distal forearm. The relevance of changes of these sites to changes in other parts of the skeleton where age-related fractures occur is questionable. Good correlations have sometimes been demonstrated between the different measurements of bone mass, but to predict with confidence what is happening at a distant site the correlation coefficient would need to be greater than 0.9, which it is not. Changes with ageing that are measured at one site may not reflect what is happening at another site or to the skeleton as a whole.

Cross-sectional data reflect what is happening in the population. However, bone mass varies considerably between subjects. Trabecular volume may vary by 25% at any one age and rates of change in bone mass may also differ according to the anatomical location. The menopause has no set time of onset and this makes it difficult to determine its effects on the onset and rate of loss of bone

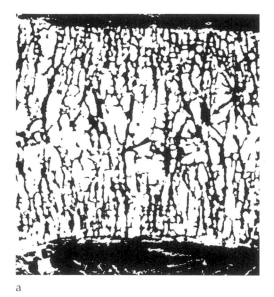

a

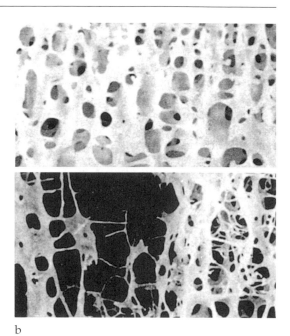

b

Figure 2.6   (a) With age there is a loss of horizontal trabeculae of the vertebrae with relative accentuation of the vertical trabecular pattern. (b) The thinning of trabecular is shown in scanning electron micrographs of normal and osteoporotic bone. Figure 2.6 (b) is reproduced with permission from The National Osteoporosis Society.

cent of the compressive strength of normal compact bone and 70% of the strength of normal trabecular bone is related to its mass. In vitro experiments have shown strength to decline with age.[19]

The strength of bone is not purely related to the quantity of mineral, but to its internal architecture. Its structure is such that it efficiently resists bending, compressive and tortional forces. The pattern of bone loss may in fact be more important than the size of bone loss in influencing the changes in its fragility. The vertical trabeculae in the spine are important for resisting the compressive forces. They are thicker and stronger than the horizontally orientated trabeculae, which brace them laterally. However, with ageing and osteoporosis, trabecular bone mass is reduced (see Figure 2.6).

Trabecular bone loss can occur in two ways. There may be generalized thinning of the trabeculae with relative preservation of bone structure, or there may be erosion through the trabeculae leading to greater disruption of structure and reduction in strength because of loss of connectivity. Thinned trabeculae have the potential to recover during a period of net bone gain, whereas eroded and perforated trabeculae may not. Successive waves of bone loss and partial recovery however will lead to some thin, unbraced trabeculae which fracture and lose connectedness. With ageing there is an increasing number of such microfractures (see Figure 2.7). They are usually repaired, but any abnormality of resorption or formation will impair healing. An impairment of this healing process may be an unwanted effect of reducing bone resorption with an agent such

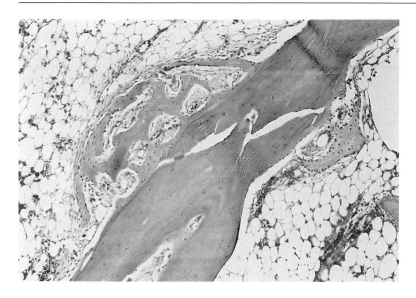

Figure 2.7   A trabecular microfracture with callus formation.

as a bisphosphonate in an attempt to treat osteoporosis and is why the long-term effect of these drugs on fracture risk needs to be evaluated.

It is principally the calcium content that is being assessed when bone mass is measured. It must not be forgotten, however, that the calcium is deposited on a matrix composed predominantly of collagen and proteoglycan so primary changes of this matrix with ageing will have a secondary effect on bone mass. Skin thickness declines with age (see Figure 2.8) and blood vessels walls, of which collagen is an important constituent, become more fragile. Bone matrix collagen may also weaken with age.

BONE ANATOMY

There is a positive relationship between body height and hip fracture. It has been suggested that the trend to increased body height in

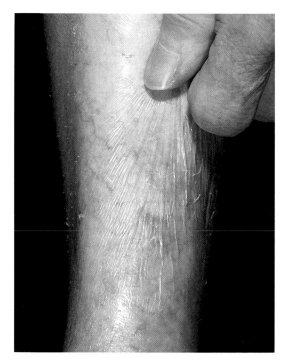

Figure 2.8   With age skin becomes thinned.

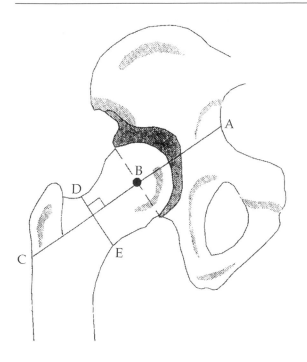

Figure 2.9   Right hip joint.
AC = hip axis length;
BC = femoral length;
DE = femoral width.

developed countries, presumably due to better childhood nutrition, may be one of the factors explaining the secular increase in the incidence of hip fracture. Similarly, an increase in hip axis length during the last 40 years may account for the age-adjusted increase in hip fractures.[20] O'Neill and colleagues compared measurements of the proximal femur for UK women aged 55–69 over a 36-year period and found changes which might explain up to one-third of the increases in incidence of hip fracture during this period (see Figure 2.9).[21]

TRAUMA

The trauma that precipitates an osteoporotic fracture is nearly always a fall, although occasionally the fall follows a cracking noise from the hip. With vertebral collapse fractures, there may be no history whatsoever of trauma,

or the force causing the collapse may be merely muscular. An epileptic fit, which sometimes complicates hypoglycaemic attacks in diabetics, is sufficient. The more usual cause of an osteoporotic fracture is a fall from a standing height or less.

Falls

More than one in three elderly people will have a fall each year. Such falls lead to major injuries more frequently than in the young, the frequency rising very steeply in very elderly people.[22] The increased susceptibility of the elderly to fracture following falls is clearly exemplified by the dramatic increase in fractures of the proximal femur and of the distal radius that occurs in snowy weather compared with the minor increase of fractures of the young. The elderly are admitted to hospital more often following a fall and their mortality is much higher. Three-quarters of fatal falls in the USA occur in those over 65 years.

There are numerous causes of falls in the elderly (see Table 2.2).[23] These can be broadly divided into intrinsic and extrinsic causes, while multiple risk factors are often present. Specific diseases of the elderly are less important than the general deterioration of various organ functions with age. Balance is often impaired and can be demonstrated with measures of sway. There is progressive muscular weakness and slowness linked to the decrease in the proportion of fast-twitch anaerobic muscle fibres compared with the slow-twitch aerobic muscle fibres. Reflex responses are often impaired or absent. Vision may be impaired and spectacles not worn at all times, leading to tripping over objects that have not been seen. Bifocal spectacle lenses have caused falls: they confuse the perception of distance and lead to missing a step. Old people tend to shuffle. 'Trainer'-type shoes with thick soles and indented treads increase friction on carpets and are less suitable for indoor wear than shoes with thinner and smoother soles. In addition, the elderly may be slightly confused. All these considerations increase the risk of falling. If they do fall, the elderly are less able to break their impact because of weakness or slower reaction time and they tend to have less protective adiposity. Specific illnesses may have a role in a minority. For example, Parkinsonism, arthritis and cardiovascular disease all affect mobility and stability, while confinement to bed for intercurrent illnesses such as pneumonia is often followed by rapid deterioration in balance and co-ordination.

Reduced grip strength, reduced skin thickness, increased body sway, decreased muscle strength, inability to rise unaided from a chair and the duration of institutionalization are all measurable correlates of general frailty, which may be more important than bone density in predicting hip fracture in this age group[24], a conclusion supported by the EPIDOS study,[25] a large study of French elderly women, which found that slower gait speed, difficulty in doing tandem (heel to toe) walk and reduced visual acuity were significant and independent predictors of the risk of hip fracture in elderly mobile women.

Table 2.2   Causes of falls in the elderly

General
- Diminished postural control
- Abnormal gait
- Weakness
- Poor vision
- Slow reaction time

Specific
- Arthritis
- Cerebrovascular disease
- Parkinson's disease
- Cataracts
- Retinal degeneration
- Menière's disease
- Blackouts
    Syncope: Carotid sinus hypersensitivity (associated with giant cell arteritis)
              Cough syncope
              Micturition syncope
    Hypoglycaemia
    Postural hypotension
    Cardiac arrhythmias (Adams-Stokes attacks)
    Acute onset cerebrovascular accident or transient ischaemic attack
    Epilepsy
    Drop attacks – ? due to vertebrobasilar insufficiency
- Drugs
    Sedatives
    Hypotensive agents
    Antidiabetic drugs
- Alcohol

The environment
- Slippery surfaces
- Uneven pavements
- Loose rugs
- Poor lighting
- Bad weather
- Worn foot rubbers on walking sticks
- Tripping over pet animals, children's toys, etc.

home-living elderly subjects the hip protectors were shown to reduce the risk of fracture by more than half, although others have not had quite so much success.[36]

There is a significant risk of death following a fall. In 1982, 11 600 deaths followed falls in the USA, 70% of which occurred in the elderly. The death rate rose logarithmically over the age of 65 years.[37] Lucht[32] found a mortality rate following a fall of 1% between the age of 60 and 69 years, but 24% over the age of 90 in fallers who presented to casualty departments. Fifty-five per cent of the over-90s who sustained a fracture of the proximal femur died. Walker[38] found that the death rate following unintentional injury rose from 93 per 100 000 in the decade 65–74 years, to 625 per 100 000 in those over 85 years. The death rate per injury rose far more rapidly with age than did the injury rate itself.

A simple fall in the house thus has a significant risk of death in the elderly. It is wrong to call these falls accidents as it implies that they are ordained by fate. It is best to consider them as unintentional injuries that can and should be prevented.

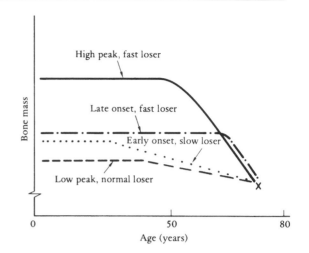

Figure 2.10   There are several different ways of developing a low bone mass, depending on the peak attained and the onset and rate of subsequent loss.

REGULATION OF BONE MASS

It is the fracture which brings the patient with osteoporosis to the doctor but the underlying cause is brittleness of bones. It is the individuals with skeletal fragility, the at-risk population, that we must identify and not just those who present with fracture. Bone mass is the major determinant of skeletal strength, although the importance of the internal architecture has been pointed out (see page 37).

The skeleton grows until the age of about 20 to 25 years, and then consolidates with accretion of mineral that accounts for about 10% of the peak adult bone mass. Following this stage, bone mass declines. The bone mass at any age following skeletal maturity depends on the peak mass that was attained and the subsequent loss. An elderly individual may have a low bone mass because of any or several of a number of processes (see Figure 2.10). Subjects may be rapid losers, this process having started either from a high peak bone mass or relatively late. They may be normal or slow losers of bone, the loss having started from a low peak mass or sooner than expected. Intermittent bursts of rapid loss are also possible. Measurements of rates of formation and resorption only tell what is happening to a patient at one point in time. They do not tell us what has happened over the previous 10 years: for this, longitudinal studies are important.

Bone mass at the menopause is the best available predictor of bone mass 20–30 years later. Peak bone mass is determined by the combination of genetic potential modified by environmental factors (such as dietary protein and calcium during the years of growth), coupled with regular exercise. Which genes and how these interact with other factors is not yet understood.

Throughout life bone is continually being formed and replaced. During growth this dynamic equilibrium is in favour of net

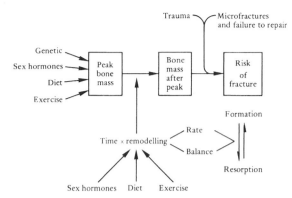

Figure 2.11 Determinants of bone mass.

loss of finer trabeculae in trabecular bone. The remodelling of cortical bone is slower than that of trabecular bone: 3% per annum compared with 30% per annum for vertebral trabecular bone and 60% per annum for iliac crest trabecular bone. Thus, changes in bone mass usually occur more rapidly in the latter.

The determinants of bone mass will therefore be discussed as first, those influencing peak mass and secondly, those influencing subsequent loss (see Figure 2.11).

Attaining peak bone mass

Peak bone mass is determined by the genetic potential as modified by:

- nutrition
- exercise
- hormonal status
- disease.

Genetic potential

Genetic factors account for 75–80% of the interindividual variation in bone mass. This has been shown in twin and family studies.

It is difficult to separate the roles of heredity and of the environment in the determination of peak bone mass. Studies of twins[39] have shown less variation of bone mass between monozygotic pairs than dyzygotic pairs, but with ageing the differences between co-twins widened. This would suggest that in youth genetic factors were predominant and environmental factors became important later, but environmental factors in utero, such as inequality of placental nutrition in twins, can also affect fetal growth. Body weight at one year of age but not weight at birth was a predictor of adult bone mass.[40] Some families are large-boned and others are small-boned. Bone mass is lower in young women whose mothers had suffered osteoporotic fractures.[41]

formation, but with ageing the balance swings in favour of resorption. The extent of loss of bone mass with ageing will depend on the size and duration of this negative balance (see Figure 2.11), and is affected by genetic make-up, age, gonadal hormones, diet and exercise.

Formation and resorption are normally closely coupled, so for there to be a net loss of bone there must be a partial breakdown of the co-ordinated activity of osteoblasts and osteoclasts (see Chapter 1). In the remodelling of bone, osteoblasts first remove a fine layer of surface protein, which allows the osteoclast to fix to the surface and start resorbing bone. Subsequent new bone formation will occur only on a surface that has been subject to previous osteoclastic resorption. Osteoblasts and osteoclasts are not the only cells present: there are also other lining cells and cells associated with bone vasculature which could play a part. It is at this cellular level that the imbalance between formation and resorption is occurring, resulting in the widening of the Haversian canals and increased intracortical porosity in cortical bone and an irreversible

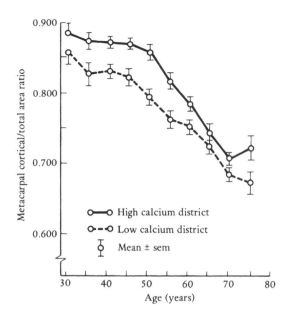

Figure 2.12 Cortical bone mass of women from the former Yugoslavia living in high versus low calcium districts.

Hypotheses which may explain this postmenopausal calcium malabsorption include a primary intestinal defect or a lack of, or relative resistance to, 1,25-dihydroxy-vitamin D_3. There are data to support and to contradict each.

Malnourished adults in the Third World, however, do not have a high incidence of osteoporosis. It is possible that they adapt to their low nutritional status by more efficient absorption and utilization of the calcium available, or that low protein diets are protective. For the maximum utilization of dietary calcium, an adequate supply of vitamin D, either in the diet, or by the exposure of the skin to sunlight, is also necessary.

Fifty per cent or more of people from black races and 5% from white races lose the intestinal enzyme lactase after weaning and this continues through childhood into adult life. Milk can give rise to diarrhoea and stomach pains in lactase-deficient children, causing them to avoid it throughout life. Moreover, elderly women compared with younger women in a New Zealand study showed a marked increase in the proportion with lactose malabsorption (60% compared with 12%). These findings may explain low calcium retention in some subjects.[64]

Factors affecting bone density after attaining peak bone mass

Bone loss is a consequence of an imbalance between formation and resorption. The net changes in bone mass can be assessed and attempts made to distinguish excessive resorption from decreased formation using techniques such as histomorphometry. These methods tell us what is happening now, but the pattern of loss may not have been uniform within an individual over time. There may have been a brief postmenopausal period of rapid bone loss but, at the time of assessment, balance between formation and resorption may have been restored. This limits the value of single point of time assessments. Patterns of loss are not uniform between individuals but no cross-sectional study has clearly shown a bimodal distribution of bone mass at any age. Many factors influencing bone loss have been identified in cross-sectional and in longitudinal studies.

Age

Ageing is the strongest associate of bone loss, as illustrated in Figure 2.5 and discussed earlier. By the age of 80 bone mass may have declined by 30% or more but there are many elderly people who do not show such a marked loss of bone mass and who do not fracture their bones. The menopause, however, is more important than age. The bone mass of women in their 50s who had a premature menopause 20 years earlier is significantly less than their age-matched (menstruating) controls, but similar to that of women in their 70s who also had their menopause 20 years earlier.[65]

Gonadal hormones

Women have less bone mass than men, and this difference increases after the menopause. Their risk of sustaining an age-related fracture is greater (see Figures 2.1 and 2.2). Albright and colleagues[1] first proposed that loss of ovarian function helped cause osteoporosis and age-related fractures in women; subsequent data have supported this. Osteoporosis develops earlier in women who have lost ovarian function through surgery or radiotherapy before the age of 45, while prospective studies have confirmed this loss of bone mass following oophorectomy and have shown that it can be prevented by oestrogen therapy.[66,67] After a natural menopause there is an acceleration of loss of bone mass which can be corrected by oestrogen therapy.[68] Oestrogen replacement improves calcium balance in postmenopausal women. Patients presenting with postmenopausal osteoporosis tend to have had a younger age of natural menopause.

Obese postmenopausal women are less likely to develop osteoporosis and vertebral crush fractures than their controls as they have higher circulating oestrone and oestradiol levels and higher peripheral conversion of androstenedione (see page 196).

Several studies have looked at whether women with postmenopausal osteoporosis have lower residual levels of sex hormones. The findings have been contradictory and have not clearly identified any major differences when compared with age-matched postmenopausal controls. Ovarian factors other than oestrogens may be important as loss of bone mass is greater after castration.

Supporting the lifetime role of oestrogens as determinants of bone mass are the negative associations of osteoporosis with frequency of lactation,[69] with high parity and with use of oral contraceptives and the associations of frequency of lactation and high parity with reduced incidence of age-related fractures.

The importance of the menopause in osteoporosis and the role of hormone replacement therapy are further discussed in Chapter 8.

Calcium

As discussed above, adequate calcium intake is important throughout life in maintaining bone density, but there are numerous influences which even in an apparently normal diet, reduce the absorption or increase the urinary excretion of dietary calcium and no simplistic equation such as 'more calcium = less osteoporosis' exists.

Exercise

With advancing age, muscle mass, bone mass and physical activity all decline. Loss of bone mass is a well recognized complication of immobility, whether as a consequence of fracture, paralysis or voluntary bed-rest,[55,70] and both young and old can be affected. The importance of weight-bearing rather than just activity has been demonstrated by the effect of space flight.[54] The increased loss of bone can be measured by increased urinary and faecal calcium excretion or by decrease in bone density. Weight-bearing bones are those most affected: up to 4% per month of the bone mass measured at trabecular sites can be lost during the initial phase of bed-rest. The loss of calcium from the whole skeleton, however, is much less (0.5% per month). The rate of bone loss reaches a new steady state after about six months of rest, while with restoration of mobility there is remineralization but this is slow and sometimes incomplete.[70] At all ages, physical activity helps maintain bone mineral content.[71]

73. Baker MR, McDonnell H, Peacock M et al. Plasma 25-hydroxy vitamin-D concentration in patients with fracture of the femoral neck. *Br Med J* (1979), i:589.

74. Tilyard MW, Spears FS, Thomson J et al. Treatment of post menopausal osteoporosis with calcitriol or calcium. *N Engl J Med* (1992), **326**: 357–62.

75. Chapuy MC, Arlot ME, Delmas PD et al. Effect of calcium and cholecalciferol treatment for three years on hip fractures in elderly women. *Br Med J* (1994), **308**: 1081–2.

76. Hodges SJ, Pilkington MJ, Stamp TCB et al. Depressed levels of circulating menaquinones in patients with osteoporotic fractures of the spine and femoral neck. *Bone* (1991), **12**: 387–9.

77. Hodges SJ, Vergnaud P, Akesson K et al. Circulating levels of vitamin K1 and K2 are decreased in elderly women with hip fracture. *J Bone Miner Res* (1993), **8**: 1241–5.

78. Watts NB, Harris ST, Genant HK et al. Intermittent cyclical etidronate treatment of postmenopausal osteoporosis. *N Engl J Med* (1990), **323**: 73–9.

79. Sebastian A, Harris JT, Ottaway JH et al. Improved mineral balance and skeletal metabolism in postmenopausal women treated with potassium bicarbonate. *N Engl J Med* (1994), **330**: 1776–81.

80. Simonen O, Laitenen O. Does fluoridation of drinking water prevent bone fragility and osteoporosis? *Lancet* (1985), **ii**: 432–3.

81. Jedrzejuk D, Milewicz A, Balanowski M et al. Does drinking water fluoridation increase bone strength in a young population? *Osteoporos Int* (1996), suppl 1, abstract 514: p. 212.

82. Saville PD. In: Barzal US ed. *Osteoporosis*. Grune and Stratton: New York (1970), pp. 38–46.

83. Hopper JL, Seemen E. The bone density of female twins discordant for tobacco use. *N Engl J Med* (1994), **330**: 387–92.

84. Forsen L, Bjorndal A, Bjartveit K et al. Interaction between current smoking, leanness, and physical inactivity in the prediction of hip fracture. *J Bone Miner Res* (1994), **9**: 1671–8.

85. Torgerson DJ, Campbell MK, Reid DM. Life style, environmental and medical factors influencing peak bone mass in women. *Br J Rheumatol* (1995), **34**: 620–4.

86. Holbrook TL, Barrett-Connor E. A prospective study of alcohol consumption and bone mineral density. *Br Med J* (1993), **306**: 1506–9.

87. Hernandez-Avila M, Colditz GA, Stampfer MJ et al. Caffeine, moderate alcohol intake and the risk of fractures of the hip and forearm in middle aged women. *Am J Clin Nutr* (1991), **54**: 157–62.

88 Dequeker J, Geusens P, Verstraeten A. Osteoarthrosis cases are not at risk for the development of osteoporosis. In: Christiansen C et al. eds. *Osteoporosis 1, Proceedings of the Copenhagen International Symposium*, Glostrop Hospital, Copenhagen, 1985, pp. 379–97.

89. Byers PD, Contepenni CA, Farkas TA. Post-mortem study of the hip joint. *Ann Rheum Dis* (1970), **29**: 15–31.

3 Methods of ascertainment and measurement of osteoporosis

INTRODUCTION

The choice of methods used to evaluate osteoporosis is dependent on the question being asked. Is it to assess the economic burden caused by osteoporosis-related disease? Is it to look at the morbidity in order to assess the impact on the individual and society? Is it to decide at what level of risk the individual is at of future osteoporosis and fracture and whether intervention is needed? Is it to follow the effects of treatment? Or is it to understand the pathogenesis of osteoporosis? Each of these may need a different approach to evaluating osteoporosis.

Osteoporosis usually presents as a low trauma fracture and these can be counted. The evaluation of any treatment for osteoporosis requires demonstration that fractures can be prevented. This is not possible in the individual but can be ascertained in populations. The impact of fractures can be measured economically, or by the social consequences, the medical complications, or effect on health-related quality of life. Ideally, it should be possible to identify individuals at risk before the fracture occurs. What can be measured is bone mass, which is the major determinant of bone strength (see Chapter 2), and markers of bone metabolism, which may predict future

fracture. The effect of treatment can be measured by the effect on fracture and its consequences, on bone mass or on bone metabolism assessed by biochemical markers or by histopathology. Pathogenesis can also be investigated by such measures of bone metabolism.

Osteoporosis is defined in terms of bone mass and this can be accurately and precisely measured (see page 28). Another important determinant of bone strength is its internal architecture, particularly of trabecular bone. Visual interpretation of the trabecular patterns in vertebrae or proximal femur, as seen on X-ray, and in the histology of an iliac crest biopsy are relatively crude. It is best assessed by magnetic resonance imaging at a clinically relevant site, but alternative methods such as microfocal radiography with fractal signature analysis are being developed.

The axial and appendicular skeleton, the cortical and trabecular bone, and the different sites of trabecular bone are all only loosely interdependent in the changes they show with age and other factors that affect total bone mass. Because of this variability in response throughout the skeleton, it is not possible to extrapolate directly from one site, at which a measurement is technically feasible, to another site, where age-related fractures are more common. Measurements are also constrained by the limitations, accessibility and cost of the technology available.

METHODS USING IONIZING RADIATION

Conventional radiographs give some information as to bone structure, quality and quantity. The progressive collapse of vertebrae or a fracture in a long bone can be detected and the trabecular pattern and cortical thickness can be assessed. Visual estimation of bone density is inadequate as 30% of the bone mass may be lost before osteopenia is apparent. Dynamic changes of cortical bone can be estimated by serial measurements of cortical thickness. Since radiographs reflect the radiodensity of calcium hydroxyapatite they cannot themselves distinguish between causes of osteopenia. There are, in addition, technical shortcomings which arise from sources of variability during exposure and development of the film. Various approaches have been developed in attempts to overcome these limitations.

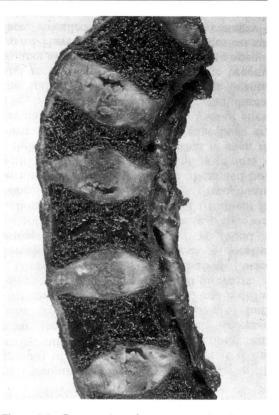

Figure 3.1 Cross-section of an osteoporotic spine showing loss of trabeculae, especially horizontally, and loss of height of vertebrae.

Vertebral bodies

With loss of bone mass the vertebral bodies become progressively radiolucent. The normal vertebral body is homogeneous in its opacity as seen on a lateral X-ray, but as vertebral osteoporosis develops there is a loss of density in the centre of the vertebral body compared with its cortical shell and at first the vertical trabecular pattern appears to be accentuated (see Figure 2.6). This is because of the differential loss of the horizontal trabeculae. With further bone loss the vertebral body appears as a hollow shell. A simple way of assessing significant vertebral bone loss is to cover the vertebral cortex and see if the trabecular core is more radio-opaque than adjacent soft tissues.

Osteoporotic vertebrae fracture and become deformed (see Figures 3.1 and 3.2), often with no history of trauma or associated acute pain. These are detected as a radiographic deformity and the problem is distinguishing a true osteoporotic vertebral fracture from other causes of vertebral deformity. If the fracture is recent, then a bone scintiscan will show increased uptake. Because it is difficult to know whether loss of vertebral height is a consequence of fracture, changes are usually described as vertebral deformities. There are two general approaches to detecting such deformities. First, by measurement of vertebral body dimensions on X-ray and using an algorithm for defining deformity. This quantitative approach is

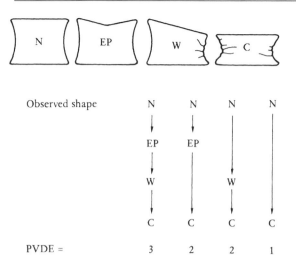

Observed shape	N	N	N	N
	↓	↓		
	EP	EP		
	↓	↓	↓	
	W		W	
	↓	↓	↓	↓
	C	C	C	C
PVDE =	3	2	2	1

Figure 3.2 Permanent vertebral body deforming events (PVDE), used to quantitate changes in the spine. The changes range from end-plate collapse (EP) to wedging (W) and crush fracture (C). N = normal.

commonly used in research studies to determine the prevalence of new vertebral deformities or to determine the incidence of vertebral deformities in therapeutic trials. The second approach is the visual inspection of vertebral shape and size on radiograph, with some criteria defining what is a deformity—a qualitative approach. This is more suitable in routine clinical practice.

The quantitative approach is based on decreases in anterior, mid or posterior vertebral heights measured as percentage changes or as multiples of standard deviation units from norms for size and shape of that vertebra. Ratios of vertebral heights either within or between vertebrae in the same individual can be used to correct for differences in skeletal size. Small deformities, such as 2 standard deviations from the mean, are not always associated with low bone mass, although two or more such deformities may be. Some deformities, especially of the thoracic spine in men, may be normal anatomic variants or may develop during growth rather than represent osteoporotic fractures.

The quantitative morphometric approach requires reference data for vertebral dimensions in a healthy population and reproducible methods. The gold standard is usually visual inspection by an expert who is best able to distinguish fractures from anomalies and assess the quality of radiographs.

The qualitative assessment is based on such an expert's opinion about what is abnormal; it is subjective and a grading is usual rather than a dichotomy of an absent or present deformity. Grading depends on whether it is a wedge, end-plate or crush deformity and on its grade of severity, which is based on the percentage decrease in vertebral body height.

There are several quantitative methods. One which is generally accepted was devised by McCloskey and colleagues for women.[1] This involves standardization of target-to-film distance at 105 cm. Thoracic films are centred on T9 and lumbar films on L3. Radiographs are positioned on a rear-illuminated digitizing grid and anterior, posterior and central heights of vertebrae are transferred to a computer for storage and comparison with subsequent radiographs. There are normal reference ranges for vertebral height and shape, and for the prevalence and incidence of vertebral deformities and an estimate of the likelihood of false positives. When making serial measurements to discover new vertebral deformities, such as when assessing the effects of preventative treatment, only those vertebrae which have been classified normal on previous films should be included.

Proximal femur

Singh index

The trabecular pattern in the proximal femur shows characteristic changes with ageing and loss of bone mass. Singh et al.[2] described a grading system based on the appearance of these changes, in which there are six grades according to the number and density of the trabecular

bone. Equations have been developed which allow the contributions of bone and of soft tissues to be differentiated. Gadolinium-153 emits photons of X-rays at both 42 and 100 keV, which are ideal photon energies for measuring bone through thick soft tissue layers. The half-life of ^{153}Gd is 242 days and the working life of the source is 12–18 months. The source is expensive and difficult to obtain. Mechanical rectilinear scans are performed and the bone mineral content is computed as grams of hydroxyapatite equivalent. Dual photon absorptiometry measures and summates the mineral content of the whole bone, both cortical and trabecular, and this reduces detection of changes in trabecular bone that occur in the spine (for example in immobilization), which although quantitatively small may have an important effect on strength.

Dual photon absorptiometry has been used successfully to demonstrate sequential changes in bone mass in the lumbar spine with age and in response to treatment. The precision of the method is good but current data suggest that measurements in an individual patient need to be as much as three years apart for changes to be meaningful.

The principal disadvantages of the method are the initial cost of the machine, and the cost of replacement of the photon source every 12–18 months and that assessments take up to 30 minutes for each patient. It is therefore not practical for routine screening of populations and has been replaced by DXA which can scan a patient in less than two minutes.

Dual X-ray absorptiometry (DXA)

Dual X-ray absorptiometry[7] has superseded other methods for estimating bone density in the spine and femoral neck (see Figure 3.5). The technology depends on delivering to the site of interest X-ray fluxes of two different frequencies, using detectors and a computer algorithm to distinguish the attenuation at each frequency level, and to deliver a measurement in terms of

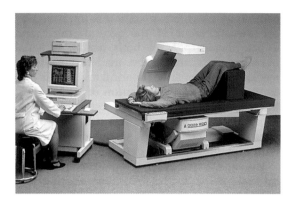

Figure 3.5 A dual energy X-ray absorptometer. (Courtesy of Vertec Scientific Ltd.)

bone mineral content. Three of the methods currently in common use are offered by Hologic, Lunar and Norland. Lunar Radiation Corporation (Livingstone, West Lothian) use a cerium-filtered spectrum which contains two peaks at 50 and 70 keV. Hologic Inc. (Waltham, Massachusetts) produce the two energies by rapidly alternating source voltages and passing the beam through a rotating calibration wheel. The beam then passes through two filters to provide the energies required. The Norland (Norland Medical Systems Inc., Fort Atkinson, Wisconsin) system is based on a samarium filter.

DXA equipment is expensive and bulky but technical development of the machines has meant that standard scans of the spine and hips can be completed faster and the latest fan beam machines can perform a scan in under one minute allowing greater throughput. This has been made possible by substituting a fan beam for the previous pencil beam, and by using a high density array of detectors instead of a single detector. At the same time the new systems produce better quality images, sufficient in most instances to make a preliminary conventional X-ray of the spine and hips unnecessary, thus saving on radiation exposure. Radiation exposure with the new machines remains low, such that the operator can stand by the machine and the patient during a scan. Nevertheless, the fan beam technique does deliver about eight times the radiation dose to the patient as does the pencil beam technique. Mechanical means of scanning the patient are gradually being replaced by improvements in computer software, with increased reliability and the ability to make further improvements. All machines give an image on the monitor screen and these can be stored in the computer and used to relocate the region of interest to be scanned so as to ensure reproducibility in serial measurements.

Technical improvements allow the deletion of metal images caused by internal orthopaedic splints and screws which might otherwise blur the images and give false high readings. Other improvements include the ability to rotate the X-ray source and the detectors through 90° in order to provide lateral scans of the lumbar vertebrae and reduce the error caused by the inclusion in anterioposterior scans of osteophytes around the disc margins and osteoarthritis of the apophyseal joints. Additionally, machines can switch to single energy mode so as to provide accurate spinal morphometry, as in assessing changes in vertebral shape. The DXA technology can be adapted to measure total body fat. Smaller DXA machines are available for measuring bone density in peripheral sites. Commercial pressures ensure both precision and accuracy and that standards are continuously being improved.

Nevertheless, the human element remains as a potential source of error. DXA machines are to osteoporosis measurement and treatment as sphygmomanometers are to blood pressure measurement and treatment, where the most reliable and reproducible results come from the use of a strictly standardized procedure. To ensure this, internationally recognized training courses and qualifications in bone density scanning are being developed. In addition, attempts are being made through the adoption of an internationally recognized reference phantom to ensure that rival systems give comparable results.[8] However, it is not possible at present to change methods of measurement when doing follow-up and serial measurements on individual patients.

For measurements of bone density at the hip, a database prepared for the (US) National Health and Examination Society (NHANES) has been accepted by the international committee for bone densitometry. International reference values for the spine are being developed but are less easy to achieve because of ethnic and other differences. There is also a need to identify one particular method of scanning as a standard by which to judge the others.

Interpreting DXA scans

The bone mineral content is the amount of bone at the site that is being measured. The bone mineral density is the bone mineral content divided by the area that is being scanned. It is an areal density, not a true density. The bone mineral density is the best measure by which to compare serial scans and follow-up. To compare individuals, results are corrected for body weight and height and expressed as a 'T' or 'Z' score[9] (see Figure 3.6).

The T score compares the findings with a young adult reference range and the Z score with an age-matched reference range. For older subjects, the T score will fall with age as bone loss is universal with ageing and it will be less than the Z score. The T score is used in the WHO definitions of osteoporosis and osteopenia, namely that osteoporosis is present if the subject has a T score in excess of 2.5 standard deviations below the mean, while values between 1 and 2.5 standard deviations below the mean are regarded as osteopenia or 'low bone mass'. That is, osteoporosis is being

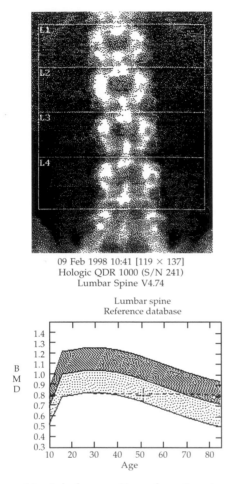

09 Feb 1998 10:41 [119 × 137]
Hologic QDR 1000 (S/N 241)
Lumbar Spine V4.74

Figure 3.6   A dual energy X-ray absorptiometry measurement of bone density at the spine.

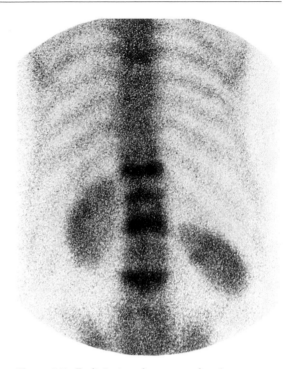

Figure 3.7   Radioisotope bone scan showing increased tracer uptake in several osteoporotic collapsed vertebrae.

Quantitative computerized tomography (CT)

defined as an absolute reduction in bone mass whether related to age or not. These definitions are useful in defining the size of the problem in epidemiological studies of populations.

The principal uses of bone densitometry are to diagnose osteoporosis or assess risk of future fracture, and in these cases the results are being compared against a normal database. When used to monitor the effects of treatment in an individual patient the errors of the method must be taken into account. Repeat scans will not give a reliable indication of response in less than a year.

Computerized X-ray tomography (CT) can be adapted to quantify bone mineral content.[10] Precise three-dimensional anatomical localization of the bone to be measured is possible and cortical bone can be measured separately from from trabecular bone. The method has a high reproducibility, with an error of 1–3%, but requires a demanding technique. Accurate measurements have been made of the tibia and femoral shaft, but the accuracy is reduced in the assessment of vertebrae and its usefulness for identifying osteoporosis at this site is limited because of difficulty in discriminating attenuation by soft tissues from attenuation by vertebral bones. The increase in marrow fat with ageing, with its low attenuation, is one important factor. The radiation dose is more

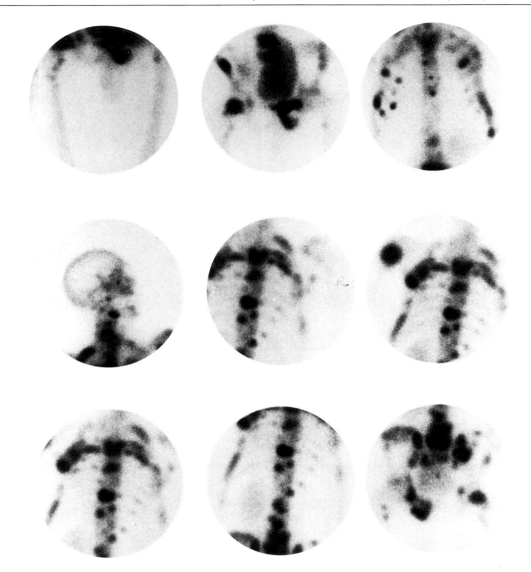

Figure 3.8 Radioisotope bone scan showing several regions of increased uptake including in the spine due to metastases.

than a hundred times that of DXA (more than 200 m rem) and the cost of the equipment is very high. This method is only a realistic proposition where existing routine CT equipment can be adapted.

Radioisotope scanning

Radioisotope scanning provides a functional assessment of bone.[11] Bone-seeking technetium-labelled bisphosphonates are used, which are adsorbed to the calcium of the hydroxyapatite crystal and give an indication both of osteoblastic activity and of skeletal vascularity. Metabolic bone disease can result in a generalized increased uptake and osteoporosis can sometimes give a 'washed out' appearance. Such changes are, however, nonspecific and are vulnerable to errors of subjective assessment. Localized areas of increased activity are seen in Paget's disease using this method, and multiple lesions of metastatic cancer can readily be demonstrated. Osteomalacia can produce focal abnormalities, typically in the ribs, while osteoporotic vertebral collapse results in a localized intense linear pattern of uptake that fades over about one year (see Figure 3.7). This picture is not specific for osteoporosis, but this is the likely diagnosis if the scan fails to show any other lesions (see Figure 3.8). Radioisotope scanning is therefore of more use in the differential diagnosis of osteoporosis than in its assessment.

Neutron activation analysis

This method allows an estimation of total body calcium content and is thus a measure of total bone.[12,13] The only other method for determining total bone mass is by an adaptation of dual energy X-ray absorptiometry. Neutron activation analysis can also be used to determine local bone mass. It is a research tool and now seldom used.

Neutron bombardment of the stable isotope ^{48}Ca, which forms 0.18% of the element, converts it to radioactive ^{49}Ca, which decays with a half-life of 8.8 minutes, emitting gamma rays. This emission is a measure of calcium content. The whole body can be bombarded with neutrons in vivo and a measurement of total calcium content, and hence skeletal mass, obtained.

The large radiation dose and the high cost of this method restrict it to a few centres with the necessary equipment. Total body calcium is higher in men than in women and is less in postmenopausal women than in premenopausal women. The fall in bone mass in postmenopausal women, as well as in rheumatoid arthritis sufferers (particularly those being treated with corticosteroids), has been confirmed and small increases caused by calcitonin or anabolic steroid treatment have been detected.

METHODS NOT USING IONIZING RADIATION

Body measurements

In the early stages of osteoporosis of the spine it is possible to measure the gradual shrinkage in height which takes place. As the erect young body gradually changes into the bent old person, there is a steady shrinkage in height which is probably part of the normal process of ageing (see Figure 3.9). It reflects both intervertebral disc narrowing and loss of vertebral body height. The changes are small, but for the whole trunk they may amount to a shrinkage of 3 mm or more per annum. This shrinkage is modulated by the circadian variation in truncal or stem height reflecting the different degrees of hydration of the discs with time of day, whereby most of us are up to 1 cm taller on rising than we were at the end of the previous day. Stem height is, however, stable in the afternoon by which time virtually all circadian shrinkage has taken place.

In severely osteoporotic subjects stem height shrinkage over the course of one year may be quite dramatic, up to 10 cm, but it is not a linear process with time (see Figure 3.10). In addition to the 'normal' shrinkage, there is an initial rapid acceleration which levels off later, probably when the rib margins begin to impact on the pelvis. There is an obvious danger in using the patient as own control. At point A in Figure 3.10, with few exceptions, the observer does not know whether the

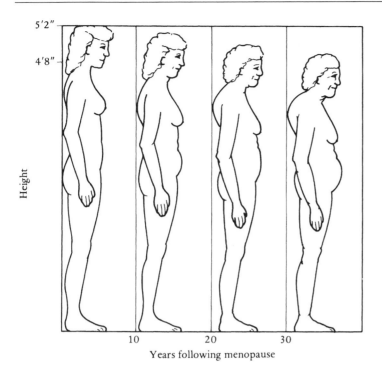

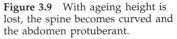

Figure 3.9   With ageing height is lost, the spine becomes curved and the abdomen protuberant.

shrinkage will occur. At point B the previous rate of shrinkage has been established, but any treatment given at this point will seem to cure the patient in that little or no further shrinkage can take place. Added to this is the difficulty of accurately measuring stem height in a subject with a dorsal kyphosis.

Nevertheless, the method is useful in comparing groups of subjects at risk of developing osteoporosis (because of corticosteroid therapy, for example), where one group is being additionally treated to prevent osteoporosis and the other is not. The method requires the subject to be seated on a standard hard-surface stool against a wall-mounted scale with a rectangular rider to measure the crown-to-rump distance. Care must be taken to ensure that clenching the buttock muscles does not introduce an error.

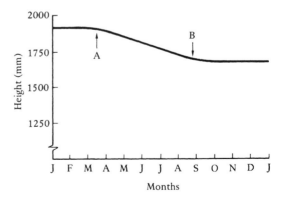

Figure 3.10   Schematic representation of stem height loss in 'active' spinal osteoporosis.

The method can be made more accurate by putting an orthopaedic X-ray ruler alongside the patient and taking a narrow beam X-ray at the stool surface and at the height of the predetermined skin mark, raising both beam and screen together in a rectilinear fashion to avoid parallax. Only a straight segment from the lower thoracic spine to L5 needs to be scanned. Changes of 2 mm or less can be discerned and the circadian variation clearly followed.[14]

Magnetic resonance imaging (MRI)

Magnetic resonance micro-tomographic imaging has emerged as a promising method of analysing trabecular structure and connectivity. Spatial resolution obtained is not yet as good a as the best X-ray-based micro-tomography, but the method has the great advantage of being non-ionizing. It promises to solve some of the clinical observations, such as the tendency of vertebrae to collapse in corticosteroid-treated subjects at higher bone densities than in subjects with age-related bone loss of similar degrees.[15]

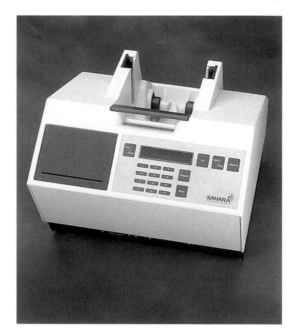

Figure 3.11   An ultrasound machine that takes measurements at the calcaneus. (Courtesy of Vertec Scientific Ltd.)

Ultrasonic bone analysis

Ultrasonic methods have been extensively researched in the hope that they will provide a non-ionizing method of assessing bone density and perhaps reveal something about bone strength. The apparatus is portable (see Figure 3.11) and several do not require immersion of the part studied. Measurements are quick and relatively cheap. Some machines provide an image of the part being studied. Bones covered with minimal soft tissue are measured, most commonly the os calcis or the patella. Two sorts of measurement can be made: speed of sound (SOS) and bone ultrasound attenuation (BUA). In a longitudinal study differential changes in the two methods after one year suggested that SOS was a better indicator of bone strength.[16]

Ultrasound measurement of the os calcis was as good as DXA measurement of bone mineral density in predicting femoral neck fracture in one large study[17] of institutionalized elderly women, but so far has not been shown to be of value for this purpose in perimenopausal women or in men. The method has been proposed as useful for preliminary screening of populations. However, the low correlation between different ultrasound machines limits its applicability. Ultrasound measurements have at present no agreed minimum and maximum values beyond which osteoporosis can be confidently diagnosed or excluded and there is at present no good evidence that it can be used to monitor the effects of treatment. Also, there is as yet no standardization or cross-calibration of the numerous types of machines and sites measured. Nevertheless, the technique is advancing rapidly. If some of these problems can be overcome the convenience of the method could lead it to become an indicator of whether more comprehensive assessment by DXA is required.

Bone biopsy

Bone biopsies are taken full thickness through the wing of the ilium into the space under the iliacus muscle to give a cylinder of bone of uniform 5 mm diameter size consisting of cortex–medulla–cortex. Up to four serial biopsies can be taken.

Indications

Bone biopsy may be indicated for diagnosis or assessment of treatment in osteomalacia, osteoporosis, hyperparathyroidism and Paget's disease, as well as in secondary invasion of bone where cancer is suspected. In the latter, X-ray films and bone scans can be used as a guide to the most likely site to pick up histologically recognizable evidence. The technique has been used in research to follow the density, compression strength and histological appearance of bone under treatment such as with fluoride.

Preparation of the patient and tetracycline labelling

Preliminaries include an X-ray of the ilium to be biopsied, a bone scan if cancer is suspected and the administration of a tetracycline to identify calcification fronts. Tetracyclines bind to newly deposited bone mineral and can be identified under fluorescence microscopy. This distinguishes between the accumulation of osteoid due to delayed mineralization or to increased synthesis. A double tetracycline label enables the rate of bone formation to be assessed. Protocols vary, but an established one[18] is as follows:

1) 250 mg of oxytetracycline three times per day for three days.
2) No medication for 12 days.
3) Second identical three-day course of oxytetracycline.
4) Biopsy three days later (which allows for good fixation of the second tetracycline label).

Technique of bone biopsy

A core of at least 5 mm diameter is obtained: the 3 mm cores obtained by Jamshedi needles are inadequate for histomorphometric analysis. The Stanmore bone biopsy assembly exemplifies the trocars available and is shown in Figure 3.12. There is an outer toothed cannula which surrounds an inner trephine-tipped cannula, within which there is an blunt-nosed obdurator.

With careful local anaesthesia the biopsy may be performed as an out-patient procedure, usually under intravenous diazepam amnesia. An overnight stay may be required by the elderly. The ideal site is 4 cm posterior and inferior to the anterior superior iliac spine (see Figure 3.13). A small incision is made through the skin and blunt dissection is used through muscle down to the periosteum under local anaesthesia with 10 ml of 1% lignocaine with adrenaline 1 in 200 000 to improve haemostasis. The whole assembly is pushed down to the bone, the teeth of the outer cannula lock on to the bone, the obdurator is withdrawn and the inner (trephine) cannula is twisted and advanced until it 'gives' when it has penetrated the distal cortex. It sometimes helps to trickle lignocaine down the inner cannula to anaesthetize the periosteum more

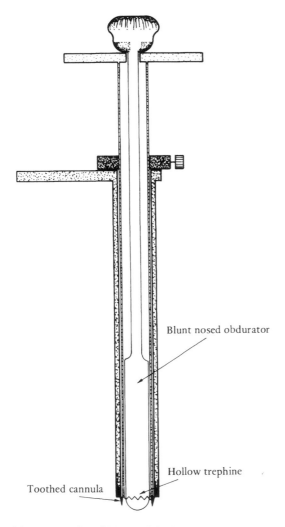

Figure 3.12 Royal National Orthopaedic Hospital (Stanmore) bone biopsy set.

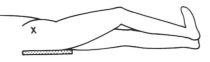

Figure 3.13 The patient should be lying, but with the side to be biopsied slightly raised by a small cushion beneath the buttock. The site is 4 cm posterior and inferior to the anterior superior iliac spine.

made of the ease with which the bone is penetrated, which can vary from very soft in severe osteoporosis to rock-hard in a young normal man.

Preparation of the specimen

This procedure is followed to prepare the specimen:

1) The core of the bone is fixed either in 10% buffered neutral formalin or, if tetracycline-labelled, in 70% ethanol (to preserve the label).
2) Once fixed, the biopsy sample can be divided into two parts longitudinally, using a heavy knife or a small fine-toothed saw, to allow the preparation of both decalcified and undecalcified specimens.
3) Decalcification in acid, such as nitric acid, eliminates the osteoid/mineralized bone interface, obscures the mineralization front and disrupts the lining cells. More information can be obtained from undecalcified sections, the quality of which is improved by resin embedding.
4) For this, the core must be dehydrated and infiltrated with methyl methacrylate. Sections of between 5 and 10 μm thick can then be obtained with a heavy sledge microtome.
5) Sections are stained with haematoxylin and eosin or by the Von Kossa silver

effectively. A stop-cuff clamped to the trephine prevents it advancing too far into the iliac fossa. The trephine is withdrawn and the specimen is expelled by the obdurator. An intact core is needed for histomorphometric analysis (see Figure 3.14). A note should be

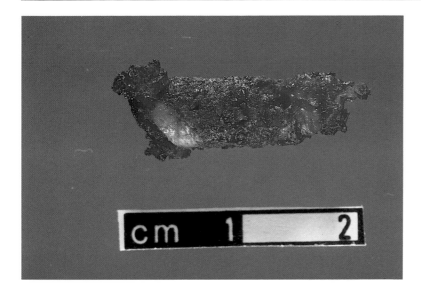

Figure 3.14 Bone core from transiliac biopsy.

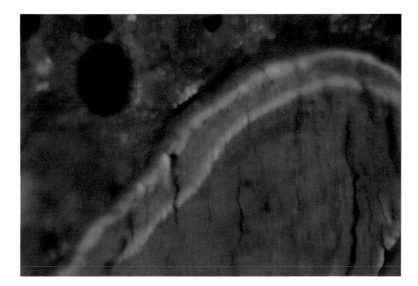

Figure 3.15 A bone biopsy that has been double tetracycline-labelled, showing the calcification fronts at the time of each administration of tetracycline.

method, which stains calcium phosphate black and osteoid red or purple. Some prefer to use a Goldner stain or modified trichrome stains for osteoid.

6) The tetracycline is visualized by fluorescence microscopy (see Figure 3.15).

Information gained

Osteoporosis is defined as a decreased mass of normally mineralized bone, that is, by histological criteria. The radiological appearance of osteoporosis and osteomalacia are often indistinguishable, and biopsy is the only absolute way of identifying the mineralization defect of osteomalacia. Biopsy can also be diagnostic in other generalized metabolic bone diseases and in cancer.

Histomorphometry, the objective measurement of the histological appearance of the bone biopsy, has developed over the last 20 years and about 50 directly measured or derived indices have been introduced.[18,19] In particular, histomorphometry allows the measurement of the amount of mineralized bone present, both cortical and trabecular, the relative amount of osteoid, and the rates of bone formation and resorption. The connectedness of the trabeculae can also be evaluated. The most useful measurements are listed in Table 3.1.[18]

A micrometer eyepiece or ocular grid can be used to measure widths and to count points of juxtaposition of histological features, with markers on the grid to estimate volumes. More sophisticated semi-automatic and automatic image analysers are available, although they are expensive. Bone collagen is normally deposited as parallel fibres of uniform diameter which can be seen under polarizing microscopy. But with increased rates of skeletal collagen synthesis there is a woven appearance of variously sized and arranged fibres.

Histomorphometry has shown the heterogeneity of osteoporosis. Some subjects show low bone turnover with formation less than resorption; others, about 10%, show accelerated turnover with resorption greater than formation; and yet others, who perhaps started with a low bone mass, show a normal rate of bone turnover. However, this assessment is made at a single time point and cannot tell us what has happened previously or exclude the possibility of sampling errors in subjects where turnover is 'quiet' in one bone site, yet 'active' in another.

Using histomorphometry, Meunier and colleagues[20] have shown that trabecular bone volume may vary widely between adjacent bone biopsies from the same individual and changes with treatment must be greater than

Table 3.1 Histomorphometric measurements

- **Trabecular bone mass**
  Trabecular bone volume (%)
  Trabecular width (μm)

- **Cortical bone mass**
  Cortical bone volume (%)
  Mean cortical widths (μm)
  Cortical porosity (%)

- **Osteoid**
  Trabecular osteoid surface (%)
  Osteoid seam width (μm)
  Trabecular osteoid volume (%)

- **Osteoblast activity**
  Trabecular osteoblastic osteoid (%)

- **Resorption**
  Trabecular resorption surface (%)
  Osteoclastic resorptive surface (%)
  Osteoclasts/mm^2 medullary space
  Osteoclasts/mm^2 trabecular area

- **Formation**
  Trabecular bone surface tetracycline-labelled (%)
  Osteoid tetracycline-labelled (%)
  Calcification rate (μm/day)
  Bone formation rate (μm/day)
  Mineralization lag time (days)

29% to be significant (a smaller percentage change is applicable if a group of 10 or more patients is studied). This limits this technique for serial studies. Histomorphometry is the most direct way of assessing the kinetics of formation and resorption. However, biochemical indices are proving to be as useful and less invasive. As a result, bone biopsy is less often indicated.

Calcium balance

Determining calcium balance by the careful assessment of calcium intake and excretion[21] is laborious and not suitable for the study of

Table 3.2 Main biochemical changes in bone disease

	Plasma			Urine	
	Calcium	*Phosphate*	*Alkaline phosphatase*	*Calcium*	*Hydroxyproline*
Osteoporosis	N	N	N	N	N
Osteomalacia	N or ↓	N or ↓	N or ↑	↓	N or ↑
Paget's disease	N	N	↑	N	↑
Primary hyperparathyroidism (with bone involvement)	↑	↓	↑	↑	↑

↑ = increase; ↓ = decrease

large numbers of subjects, but has established the optimum intake of calcium to maintain neutral balance and has demonstrated the steady net loss of calcium in the elderly. Balance studies are too vulnerable to error for the assessment of therapies for osteoporosis, except in specialized centres thoroughly accustomed to the techniques.

Clinical laboratory investigations

Laboratory tests are used in the assessment of bone turnover, in the diagnosis of the underlying cause of osteoporosis and in the differential diagnosis of other bone diseases. The basic indices of bone metabolism are the serum calcium, phosphate and alkaline phosphatase concentrations (see Table 3.2) supplemented by the more recent markers of bone formation and resorption.[22]

For assessing bone resorption there are available urinary fasting morning calcium, urinary hydroxyproline, urinary pyridinoline and deoxypyridinoline cross-links of collagen, urinary hydroxylysine glycosides and serum tartrate-resistant acid phosphatase. For assessing the rate of bone formation, circulating levels of serum bone alkaline phosphatase, serum osteocalcin and serum procollagen

Type I C-terminal propeptide can be employed. Urinary fasting collagen cross-links and the phosphatases can be effectively measured by ELISA immunoassay.

Problems that arise with biochemical markers of bone metabolism are that several are nonspecific, that there are idiosyncratic changes, there is often diurnal variation and that it is at present difficult to compare measures of formation, which are serum markers, with measures of resorption that are principally urine markers.

Calcium

The serum calcium is normal in osteoporosis, and hypercalcaemia points to malignancy or hyperparathyroidism (see Chapter 5). Hypocalcaemia may be found in osteomalacia, although calcium levels are often within the low normal range. There is a slight fall in total serum calcium with ageing, but the level of ionized calcium is unchanged. The serum calcium is largely protein-bound, mainly to albumin, and it is the bound fraction which falls with age. Because of this, it is necessary to measure the serum albumin routinely in order to correct the serum calcium levels for albumin concentration.

Phosphate

The serum phosphate level is normal in osteoporosis. It may be low in the elderly, in osteomalacia or in primary hyperparathyroidism and chronic diarrhoea. The excessive use of aluminium hydroxide will also lower it. It is increased in renal failure.

Markers of bone formation

Alkaline phosphatase

All living and dividing cells contain phosphatases which are released into the plasma on cell death or in situations of rapid cell turnover. Phosphatases have in the past been measured by the rate of hydrolysis of chromogenic esterphosphates at various pHs as regulated by the buffer system employed. At a lower pH 'acid' phosphatases are measured. A higher pH detects 'alkaline' phosphatases. More recently ELISA immunoassay has given better results. All causes of generalized inflammation, including pneumonia or active rheumatoid arthritis, will cause some increase in circulating levels of alkaline phosphatase and, as such, it acts as an acute phase indicator. The most important source, however, is hepatic alkaline phosphatase, so much so that blood levels of alkaline phosphatase are more sensitive to hepatocellular disease than to any other condition.

A normal blood level of alkaline phosphatase is up to 92 IU/litre in adults, but smaller rises above this level are common in many illnesses and have little significance. In children, higher levels are found, reflecting the increased cell turnover, both of hepatocytes and osteoblasts, due to growth. Increases in the hepatic fraction can be identified by looking at the isoenzymes or parallel changes in other hepatic enzymes, e.g. γ-glutamyl transferase or 5-nucleotidase.

In bone, an alkaline phosphatase is secreted by osteoblasts and is a marker of bone formation (see Chapter 1). It differs from the liver isoenzyme in post-translational glycosylation. It can be assayed separately. It is increased by about 20% in the menopause compared with that of premenopausal controls and continues to rise with ageing. It falls with oestrogen replacement therapy.[23] These changes are usually within the normal range of most laboratories. High levels of serum alkaline phosphatase (four times the upper level of normal or more) are rarely of bony origin and where they do occur are caused by severe, extensive and active Paget's disease. Moderate elevations of the serum alkaline phosphatase (bone isoenzyme), of up to two or three times normal, occur in hyperparathyroidism and in secondary invasion of bone by cancer (though it is not elevated in myeloma). Moderate elevation is also seen in osteomalacia.

Serum alkaline phosphatase is normal in osteoporosis but even here there are exceptions, including the osteoporosis of acute hyperparathyroidism, after recent vertebral or other fracture, and of course if there is concomitant liver disease. However, parallel studies of bone histology and biochemistry and response to vitamin D have made it clear that low-grade osteomalacia may coexist with osteoporosis in old people despite near normal blood biochemistry.

Osteocalcin

Osteocalcin, also known as bone Gla-protein (BGP), is a 5800 dalton-sized peptide containing γ-carboxyglutamic acid, the formation of which is vitamin K-dependent (see Chapter 1). It is a major protein component of bone matrix. It is predominantly synthesized by osteoblasts and serum levels reflect their activity. The form that is released from bone matrix during degradation is not complete and the antiserum used in the radioimmunoassay identifies only that released by osteoblasts. There is a small circadian rhythm and day-to-day variation. Serum osteocalcin correlates with skeletal growth at puberty and is increased in various conditions where there is increased bone turnover. It is a specific marker of bone formation.[24]

Procollagen 1 extension peptides

During the formation of collagen fibrils the extension peptides are cleared from procollagen and the terminal (PINP) and carboxyterminal peptides can be measured in the serum. They are a marker of bone formation but there are non-osseous sources.

Markers of bone resorption

Urinary hydroxyproline

Hydroxyproline forms about 13% of the amino acid content of collagen. It is formed by the post-translational hydroxylation of proline, released during degradation of collagen and cannot be reutilized. Urinary hydroxyproline is predominantly from the degradation of collagen and about half is derived from bone. Urinary hydroxyproline is therefore used as a marker of bone resorption. It is however highly metabolized before excretion, and because of this and the nonbony sources it is not a very good marker of bone resorption.

Urinary hydroxylysine glycosides

Hydroxylysine is another amino acid specific to collagen that is a potential sensitive marker of bone resorption.

Plasma tartrate-resistant acid phosphatase (TRAP)

Acid phosphatase is produced by bone, prostate, platelets, erythrocytes and the spleen. There are numerous isoforms, and bone acid phosphatase is resistant to L(+)-tartrate. It is released from osteoclasts during bone resorption. Improved assays are being developed and its usefulness is still being evaluated.

Collagen cross-links

Collagen molecules are stabilized by the post-translational formation of covalent pyridinium cross-links between various polypeptides. These are either pyridinoline (Pyd) found in a variety of tissues including bone and cartilage, and deoxypyridinoline (D-Pd) which is specific to bone. The collagen molecules form fibrils, are mineralized and remain part of bone for many years. During osteoclastic bone resorption these cross-links are released into the circulation and excreted in the urine as free pyridinoline (free Pyd) or free deoxypyridinoline (free D-Pd) or bound to Type 1 collagen fragments, linked to the C-terminal (CTX) or N-terminal (NTX) telopeptides. The total amount of urinary pyridinium cross-links (free and peptide-bound Pyd and D-Pd) can be measured by high performance liquid chromatography, but immunoassays have been developed for possible clinical use based on antibodies against free Pyd and, or free D-Pd or against peptides in the cross-link (CTX and NTX assays). As different components of the cross-links are being recognized in these assays, results may have different clinical relevance and each method needs to be evaluated in various metabolic bone diseases.

Collagen cross-links show a circadian rhythm and collection should be standardized: the first or second morning void of urine should be used. They are increased in various conditions characterized by increased bone turnover.[25,26] They are reduced by antiresorptive drug therapy, such as alendronate.[27]

Use of bone markers

High bone turnover is associated with a fast rate of postmenopausal bone loss. Markers may be useful in identifying those women most at risk of osteoporotic fracture in combination with a bone density measurement, as increased levels of markers of bone resorption are associated with increased risk of vertebral and hip fracture independent of bone mass.[28] As bone markers fall rapidly with effective therapy[27] they may be useful in monitoring response and compliance.

Other assessments of hormones regulating bone metabolism

Calcium-regulating hormones can be assayed but the methods often differ from laboratory to laboratory as does the reliability of the results. They are not yet routine investigations but may be of value in the differential diagnosis of osteopenia. Low 25-hydroxy-vitamin D levels may suggest osteomalacia due to dietary deficiency, malabsorption or renal disease. Elevated immunoreactive PTH levels indicate hyperparathyroidism.

Oestrogens and gonadotrophins

Ovarian function can be assessed by measuring oestrogen or gonadotrophin levels. Follicle-stimulating hormone (FSH), and to a lesser extent luteinizing hormone (LH), rise following the menopause and the FSH:LH ratio becomes greater than 1. Most studies have found that oestrogen levels do not discriminate between postmenopausal women with and without osteoporosis.

Other investigations in the assessment of osteopenia

Low bone mass may be associated with renal, hepatic and various endocrine diseases (see Chapter 4) and these must be excluded. Renal

and hepatic function should be screened, urine should be tested for protein and sugar, and thyroid function tests performed if there is any clinical suspicion of hyperthyroidism. Elevated mean corpuscular cell volume may identify alcoholism as a factor in the development of osteoporosis or in causing a fall and breaking a bone. Plasma protein electrophoresis and other general markers of disease (erythrocyte sedimentation rate or plasma viscosity) will identify most patients with carcinomatosis, myelomatosis or osteomyelitis of the spine who present with vertebral collapse (discussed further in Chapter 5).

Fracture rates

The ultimate purpose of the study of osteoporosis is the prevention or cure of bone structural failure, that is, liability of the skeleton to fracture or crush with minimal trauma. Bone density measurements are only an indirect method of approaching this, as the increased fragility of dense bones in osteopetrosis or after fluoride intoxication reminds us. But fracture rates also depend on other factors, including exposure to trauma (see Chapter 2). Statistical methods are therefore necessary to take into account the influence of age, season, occupation and co-morbidity on the interpretation of changes in fracture rates in studies of treatment or prevention. Fracture rates are most applicable when there has already been a significant degree of bone loss and are less applicable in younger subjects where bone loss is just beginning.

The incidence of fractures is low, so for any significant effect of treatment to be demonstrated large numbers of subjects must be studied for several years. Long bone fractures are not entirely random events but are dependent on various extrinsic factors. Vertebral compression fractures are not so dependent on trauma but new vertebral fractures have an incidence in postmenopausal women of about three per 100 patient-years of observation.

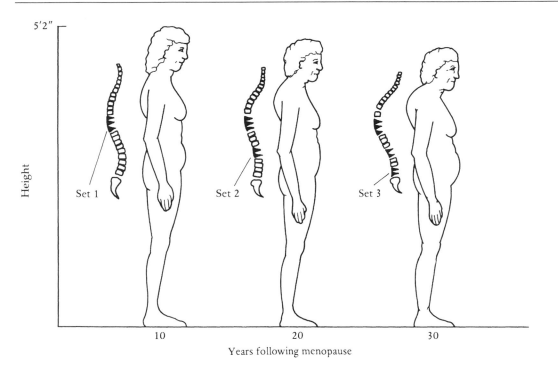

Figure 3.16 The location of vertebral fractures does not appear to be totally random, but there is a pattern with increasing age.

Changes in shape are more common and methods for assessing these have been developed (see page 59), but they do not correlate well with bone mass. They do not necessarily progress to vertebral compression fractures.

The major concern is the prevention of the fracture that carries the highest morbidity and mortality, that is, fracture of the proximal femur. It is the reduction in the incidence of this by which a treatment needs to be judged. Data exist on the effectiveness of postmenopausal hormone replacement,[29,30] alendronate[31] and of lifelong high calcium intake.[32]

There are however many difficulties in performing the large long-term studies that are required. To follow a large number of individuals for several years and maintain them on either placebo or therapy has practical and sometimes ethical problems. It is also difficult to select those who are suitable to enter such studies. Should they come from an apparently normal population, be among those who are currently recognized to be at risk of developing osteoporosis, or should they already have osteoporosis (that is, a low bone mass or have sustained an age-related fracture)? If those who have already fractured are selected, many will have a reduced risk of a subsequent fracture even without any further therapy. They may have already crushed the most susceptible vertebra (see Figure 3.16). Once a person has broken a hip, lifestyle may be altered so as to reduce the risk of further fractures independently of any treatment.

These difficulties must be met and long-term studies must be set up to establish, for instance, whether a beneficial effect of an agent on radial bone mass is paralleled by a reduction in the incidence of Colles' fractures. The value of such studies is exemplified by the elegant data from Glasgow showing the effect of hormone replacement therapy in oophorectomized women followed for 12 years or more.[33]

Postmortem and histological studies

Information on the frequency of osteoporosis, the compression strength of vertebrae and the fracture resistance of long bones can be obtained at postmortem, but such methods are limited in application because pathologists seldom investigate matters other than the immediate cause of death in the main coelomic cavities. Autopsy rates vary enormously between countries and cultures. Information can be gained from surgical specimens, for example, from the femoral neck when a fracture here has been treated by total hip replacement arthroplasty.

Table 3.3   Questions to ask of methods

1   *Is it measuring what we want?* This questions the accuracy of a method; for example, quantitative CT scanning measures bone *and* marrow fat.

2   *Is it measuring the relevant site?* The best correlation between bone mass and risk of fracture is obtained if assessed at the fracture site, or its opposite. Changes in the appendicular skeleton do not necessarily reflect the changes in the axial skeleton.

3   *Is it practical to assess large numbers of individuals?* This is important in epidemiological studies, and requires simple and inexpensive methods.

4   *Is it precise enough for longitudinal studies?* The rate of loss of bone is slow and the best methods, such as dual energy X-ray absorptiometry, cannot expect to show meaningful changes in less than one year.

5   *Is it giving any information as to the pathogenesis of osteoporosis?* Does it distinguish between increased resorption or decreased formation of bone? Radiogrammetry, histomorphometry and biochemical indices can help distinguish.

6   *Does it exclude other causes of low bone mass?* Bone biopsy and other investigations may be necessary (see Chapter 5).

WHICH METHOD TO CHOOSE

There is as yet no satisfactory method of identifying those who will fracture before the event. Reduced bone mass is one of the best predictors available of an increased risk of fracture, particularly if measured at the site of potential fracture, for instance the femoral neck or the vertebral bodies. Dual energy X-ray absorptiometry (DXA) can accurately and reproducibly assess bone mass at these sites. Not all those with low bone mass will fracture, and the debate about the clinical role of these measurements is fully reviewed in Chapter 7.

As there are various methods looking at different aspects of osteoporosis, it is important to decide what question is being asked, and to understand the weaknesses and advantages of the various methods as detailed within this chapter and in Table 3.3. Most clinicians will be limited by the methods that are available locally but at least an understanding of the problems of assessment will help them in their interpretation of the results from whatever method is used and also allow a critical analysis of the published data.

PRACTICAL POINTS

- Conventional X-rays are simple, safe, cheap and suitable for many investigations in osteoporosis. They give information as to structure and quality but not bone density.

- The mineral content of bone is best studied by dual X-ray absorptiometry (DXA).

- In early osteoporosis, the gradual shrinkage in height can be measured.

- Bone biopsy may be indicated in osteoporosis (and other bone diseases) for diagnosis or assessment of treatment.

- Bone markers help in predicting fracture risk and monitoring therapy.

- The cause of, or differential diagnosis of osteoporosis should be investigated and this includes biochemical screening, isotope scanning and bone biopsy.

REFERENCES

1. McCloskey EV, Spector TD, Eyres KS et al. The assessment of vertebral deformity: a method for use in population studies and clinical trials. *Osteoporos Int* (1993), **3**: 138–47.
2. Singh M, Nagrath AR, Malni PS. Changes in the trabecular pattern of the upper end of the femur as an index of osteoporosis. *J Bone Joint Surg [Am]* (1970), **52A**: 457–67.
3. Horsman A, Nordin C, Simpson M et al. Cortical and trabecular bone status in elderly women with femoral neck fracture. *Clin Orthop* (1982), **166**: 143–51.
4. Exton-Smith AN, Millard PH, Payne PR et al. Method of measuring quantity of bone. *Lancet* (1969), **ii**: 1153–4.
5. Barnett B, Nordin BEC. A radiological diagnosis of osteoporosis. *Clin Radiol* (1960), **11**: 166–74.
6. Glüer CC, Steiger P, Genant HK. Validity of dual-photon absorptiometry. *Radiology* (1988), **166**: 574–5.
7. Lafferty FW, Rowland DY. Correlations of dual energy X-ray absorptiometry, quantitative computed tomography, and single photon absorptiometry with spinal and non-spinal fractures. *Osteoporos Int* (1996), **6**: 407–15.
8. Pearson J, Dequeker J, Henley M et al. (The European Quantitation of Osteoporosis Study Group). European semi-anthropometric spine phantom for the calibration of bone densitometers: assessment of precision, stability and accuracy. *Osteoporos Int* (1995), **5**: 174–84.
9. Kanis JA, Devolaer J-P, Gennari C. Practical guide for the use of bone mineral measurements in the assessment of osteoporosis: position paper of the European Foundation for Osteoporosis and Bone Disease. *Osteoporos Int* (1996), **6**: 256–61.
10. Cann CE, Genant HK, Kolb FO et al. Quantitative computed tomography for prediction of vertebral fracture risk. *Bone* (1985), **6**: 1–7.
11. Alazraki N. Bone imaging by radionuclide techniques. In: Resnick D, Niwayama G eds. *Diagnosis of bone and joint disorders*. WB Saunders: Philadelphia (1981), pp. 639–78.
12. Anderson J, Osborn SB, Tomlinson RWS et al. Neutron activation analysis in man in vivo. A new technique in medical investigation. *Lancet* (1964), **ii**: 1201–5.
13. Reid DM. Measurement of bone mass by total body calcium: a review. *J R Soc Med* (1986), **79**: 33–7.
14. Dixon AS, Hawkins S, Williams C. Circadian variation in segmental vertebral height in spinal osteoporosis. In: *Osteoporosis 1, Proceedings of the Copenhagen International Symposium*, Glostrop Hospital, Copenhagen, 1985, p. 231.
15. Majumdar S, Newitt D, Mathur A et al. Magnetic resonance imaging of trabecular bone structure in the distal radius: relationship with X-ray tomographic microscopy and biomechanics.

Osteoporos Int (1996), **6**: 376–85.

16. Krieg MA, Thiebaud D, Burckhardt P. Quantitative ultrasound of bone in institutionalised elderly women: a cross sectional and longitudinal study. *Osteoporos Int* (1996), **6**: 189–95.

17. Hans D, Dargent-Molina P, Schott AM et al. Ultrasonographic heel measurements to predict fracture in elderly women: the EPIDOS study. *Lancet* (1996), **348**: 511–14.

18. Vigorita VJ. The bone biopsy protocol for evaluating osteoporosis and osteomalacia. *Am J Surg Pathol* (1984), **12**: 925–30.

19. Recker RR ed. *Bone histomorphometry: techniques and interpretation.* CRC Press: Boca Raton (1983).

20. Chavassieux PM, Arlot ME, Meunier PJ. Intersample variation in bone histomorphometry: comparison between parameter values on two contiguous bone transiliac bone biopsies. *Calcif Tissue Int* (1985), **37**: 345–50.

21. Heaney RP, Recker RR, Saville PD. Calcium balance and calcium requirements in middle-aged women. *Am J Clin Nutr* (1977), **30**: 1603–11.

22. Eastell R. Biochemical markers. In: *Spine: State of the art reviews* (1994), **8**: 155–70.

23. Christansen C, Rødbro P, Tjellesen L. Serum alkaline phosphatase during hormone treatment in early postmenopausal women. *Acta Med Scand* (1984), **216**: 11–17.

24. Lian JB, Gundberg CM. Osteocalcin: biochemical considerations and clinical applications. *Clin Orthop Rel Res* (1988), **226**: 267–91.

25. Delmas PD, Schlemmer A, Gineyts E et al. Urinary excretion of pyridinoline crosslinks correlates with bone turnover measured on iliac crest biopsy in patients with vertebral osteoporosis. *J Bone Miner Res* (1992), **6**: 639–44.

26. Delmas PD, Gineyts E, Bertholin A, Garnero P, Marchand F. Immunoassay of pyridinoline crosslink excretion in normal adults and in Paget's disease. *J Bone Miner Res* (1993), **8**: 643–8.

27. Garnero P, Shih WJ, Gineyts EB et al. Comparison of new biochemical markers of bone turnover in late postmenopausal women in response to alendronate treatment. *J Clin Endocrinol Metab* (1994), **79**: 1693–700.

28. Garnero P, Sormony-Rendu E, Chapuy M-C et al. Increased bone turnover in late postmenopausal women is a major determinant of osteoporosis. *J Bone Miner Res* (1996), **11**: 337–49.

29. Weiss NS, Ure CL, Calard JH et al. Decreased risk of fractures of the hip and lower forearm with postmenopausal estrogen. *N Engl J Med* (1980), **303**: 1195–8.

30. Kiel DP, Felson DT, Anderson JJ et al. Hip fracture and the use of estrogens in postmenopausal women. The Framingham study. *N Engl J Med* (1987), **317**: 1169–74.

31. Black DM, Cummings SR, Karpf DB. Randomised trial of effect of alendronate on risk of fracture in women with existing fractures. *Lancet* (1996), **348**: 1535–41.

32. Matkovic V, Kostial K, Simonovic I et al. Bone status and fracture rates in two regions of Yugoslavia. *Am J Clin Nutr* (1975), **32**: 361–3.

33. Lindsay R, Cosman F, Nieves JJ. Estrogen: effects and actions in osteoporosis. *Osteoporos Int* (1993), **3**: S150–2.

4 Clinical presentations and associations

GENERALIZED OSTEOPOROSIS

In generalized forms of osteoporosis all bones in the body progressively lose calcium and the supporting collagen framework of the bone. This continues until, at some point, bone structural failure occurs. It is convenient however to subdivide generalized osteoporosis into that mainly affecting cortical bone and that mainly affecting trabecular bone. The subdivision is largely artificial but has clinical significance:

- In failure of cortical bone there is usually a fracture of one of the long bones (see Figure 4.1). The fracture will be obvious and painful, will often be associated with displacement but, if correctly set, will heal normally within a normal time. The immediate clinical problem therefore is no different from that of any other fracture.
- In contrast, bone structural failure in the spine, which is mainly trabecular bone, results in wedging or crushing of vertebral bodies without displacement, sometimes without pain and with no possibility of resuming normal vertebral height. These changes result in spinal shrinkage and often unnatural curvatures (see Figure 4.2).

Bone mass reaches a peak at 35 years, following which there is a loss of both cortical and trabecular bone. This loss is greater in women who at all ages have less total bone mass than men (see Figure 2.5). The total loss of cortical bone in women may be more than four times that in men by the age of 80 years. Trabecular bone mass similarly decreases with ageing but begins earlier. By the age of 85 years women may have lost about 50% of vertebral bone compared with 20% in men. Bone loss is not uniform throughout the skeleton as there are differing proportions of cortical and trabecular bone at various sites and different factors affect their respective losses. Glucocorticoid therapy is mainly associated with trabecular loss. Bone loss can also vary between individuals. The differential loss of cortical and trabecular bone will produce a different risk of fracture at different sites depending on the ratio of cortical to trabecular bone. Two patterns of bone loss have been described, one predominantly trabecular with an early increased incidence of vertebral and Colles' fracture between the ages 50 and 65 years, and another type, characterized by both trabecular and cortical loss and associated with an increased incidence of fractures of the femoral neck, usually occurring over the age of 75 years (see Figure 2.2).

Trabecular bone predominates in the vertebral bodies and to a lesser extent in the posterior calcaneum, in the lower end of the radius, in the femoral condyles in the knee and in the intertrochanteric region of the femur.

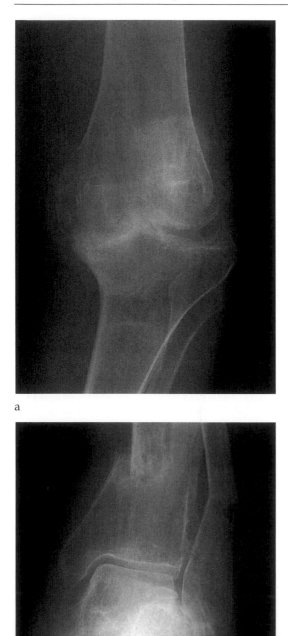

a

b

Figure 4.1
Fractures of the distal tibia and fibula (a).
Rheumatoid arthritis has caused destruction of the
lateral compartment of the knee resulting in vagus
deformity and osteoporosis (b). The resulting
abnormal stress at the ankle has resulted in failure of
the cortical bone and fracture.

Elsewhere, however, cortical bone predominates and overall constitutes 80% of the total
skeleton. Trabecular bone, because of its large
and readily available surface area, is much
more metabolically active, and it is in trabecular bone that changes in bone mass occur first
and are most marked in response to immobility. Cortical bone also reacts, but usually more
slowly and to a lesser extent. Thus, in chronic
causes of net bone resorption osteoporosis of
cortical bone will eventually occur. The width
of the cortex will shrink gradually and it will
increase in porosity, but should healing take
place it will largely restore the original cortical
architecture since the foundation on which to
rebuild bone remains. In contrast, trabecular
bone will suffer most as there is a selective
irreversible loss of trabeculae, the processes of
thinning or perforation leading to loss of
connectivity of trabeculae, so that with recovery only those trabeculae which escaped dissolution will be in a position to be reinforced. On
X-ray this change will appear as bone that has
regained overall density but shows a very
coarse trabecular pattern which does not
necessarily restore the original bone strength.

Trabecular bone fractures, especially those
which occur in the spine of elderly women, may
happen so slowly and insidiously that they are
painless and unnoticed; the patient presenting
with kyphosis or loss of height. In contrast, for
long bones to fracture there requires to be not
only bone weakness but also trauma. The
greater the degree of cortical osteoporosis, the
more trivial the trauma which can cause a
fracture. Considerations of the consequences of
cortical osteoporosis must always include those
other factors, extrinsic and intrinsic, leading to
fracture (see Chapter 2).

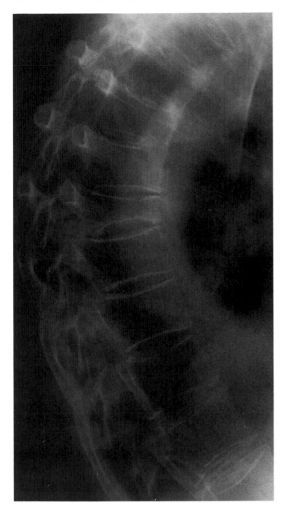

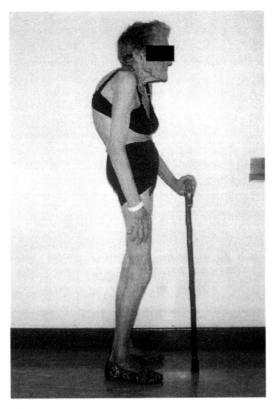

Figure 4.3
A 69 year old woman with spinal shrinkage but no history of acute pain in the back nor of trauma to the spine.

Figure 4.2
Osteoporosis of the thoracic spine with crush fracture of a vertebra. Note the marked vertical trabeculation of other vertebrae—a feature of early bone loss.

Postmenopausal and senile osteoporosis

It is convenient to distinguish clinically between 'senile' (men and women) and 'postmenopausal' (women) forms of osteoporosis but there seem to be no essential differences between them and both are often described together as 'involutional osteoporosis'.

By custom, involutional osteoporosis is that in which any known predisposing cause of osteoporosis (such as hyperthyroidism or corticosteroid therapy) can be ruled out. However, the effect of such known causes is often first revealed or most evident in those age groups in which involutional osteoporosis is most prevalent. For osteoporosis in general, the causes add up.

To recapitulate, age-related loss of bone mass is paralleled by age-related increases in fractures of bones, particularly of the distal radius, proximal humerus, femoral neck and vertebral bodies. Whereas osteoporotic fractures of the vertebral bodies may occur spontaneously and sometimes without pain (see Figure 4.3), osteoporotic fractures of the long bones are usually precipitated by a fall and are painful. What would seem a trivial fall may result in fracture, and most falls occur from standing height or less. Such falls are common in the elderly and there are many, often interrelated, causes (see Chapter 2).

Idiopathic generalized osteoporosis

Juvenile[1]

Osteoporosis is rare in childhood. Known causes are Cushing's syndrome (spontaneous or drug-induced), coeliac disease (which may also cause rickets), immobilization, juvenile polyarthritis, leukaemia, homocystinuria and osteogenesis imperfecta. There remains however a small group with idiopathic juvenile osteoporosis: less than 100 instances of this have been described. The severity of the condition varies from mild involvement of the spine alone (causing kyphosis) to severe, progressive osteoporosis with multiple fractures and deformity. The main differential diagnosis is with one of the nonfatal forms of osteogenesis imperfecta but the blue sclerae, familial predisposition, deafness and dentigenesis imperfecta of the latter sets it apart from juvenile osteoporosis.

The cause of idiopathic juvenile osteoporosis is obscure but in about half of such children the changes are reversible. The calcium balance is neutral or negative when at this age it should be positive, but without evidence of osteomalacia to suggest a disorder or deficiency of vitamin D. Whether there is a deficiency of osteoblastic activity or excessive osteoclastic activity is unclear.

Patients present with pain in the back or extremities due to fracture. Presentation can be

between the ages of four and 20 years, but usually just before puberty (though earlier in girls) and the disease remits after adolescence. Difficulty in walking and an abnormal gait are common. Examination only reveals the kyphosis and possibly bony deformities of limbs consequent upon fracture. Children with idiopathic juvenile osteoporosis may (as may children with osteogenesis imperfecta) be suspected of being 'battered babies', to the embarrassment of their parents.

There are no consistent biochemical changes, although hypercalciuria is not uncommon. The erythrocyte sedimentation rate may be elevated. X-rays of the spine reveal the multiple compressed or biconcave vertebrae and often there are metaphysial compression fractures of the long bones, in particular of the distal tibia. Sometimes there is osteoporotic new bone in the metaphyses, and also subperiostially in the pubic rami and the femoral neck. In mild disease, remodelling of the vertebrae is seen before growth ceases and the eventual height of the sufferer is not seriously reduced.

There is no known useful treatment.

Adult

Adult idiopathic generalized osteoporosis is rare. It occurs in young men or premenopausal women, in whom all investigations fail to identify a primary cause.[2,3] In women it may follow childbirth (see Figure 4.4). Some sufferers may represent the end result of idiopathic juvenile osteoporosis, and late osteogenesis imperfecta must also be considered. The presentation is with decreasing height, usually without marked kyphosis or much pain.

Men with osteoporosis[4-6]

Compared to women, men have a higher peak bone mass, do not suffer the acceleration of

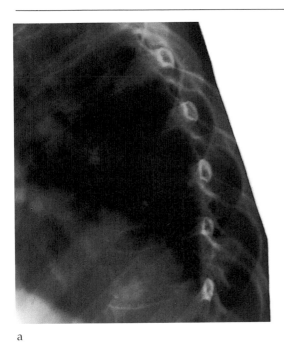

a

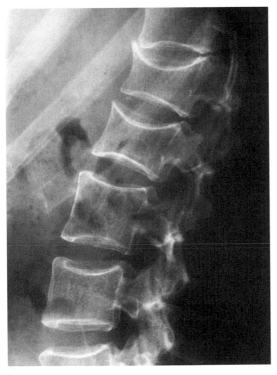

b

Figure 4.4
Postpartum osteoporosis. A 33-year-old woman who, four months after the birth of her third child, developed back pain. The X-ray shows osteopenia of the (a) thoracic and (b) lumbar spine with ballooning of the discs and wedging of the vertebrae.

bone loss associated with the menopause and on average live five years less. The incidence of osteoporosis in men is thus much less than that in women. Even so, by the age of 60 years 3% of men will have suffered an osteoporosis-related fracture rising to 8% by the age of 80 years. Hip fractures are most frequent in the eighth and ninth decades and, as in women, most are related to falls from a standing height, affect those who live alone, have a poor diet, or who through age, frailty or co-morbidity live in institutions. Hip fractures in men at this age have a high morbidity and mortality. Fall-related fractures also occur in the distal radius, proximal ulna and in the pelvis. However, in some men a fall is the result, not the cause, of the fracture, with the sufferer collapsing whilst walking in the street perhaps without any previous pain or other warning. In similar instances an X-ray to confirm the fracture has revealed an incipient stress fracture in the opposite femoral neck.

Spinal deformities are found in younger men but some of this may be developmental and not related to osteoporosis. Vertebral osteoporosis is due to secondary causes in 40–60% of men with symptomatic spinal fractures (Table 4.1). The commonest predisposing cause for a spinal crush fracture in men is corticosteroid therapy. The risk is increased by the effect of the disease for which the treatment is given, such as rheumatoid arthritis or asthma.

Primary hypogonadism is apparent in some men with osteoporosis and this also responds to androgen treatment.[7] Hypogonadism may contribute to hip fracture in elderly men,[8] whilst delayed puberty in male youths can

Table 4.1   Causes of spinal osteoporotic crush fractures in men

Cause	n	%
Primary	231	40
Secondary	351	60
Glucocorticoid therapy, Cushing's syndrome	90	15.5
Neoplastic	15	2.5
Osteogenesis imperfecta	9	1.5
Gastric surgery	13	2.2
Hypogonadism	40	7
Thyroid excess	11	1.9
Heparin treatment and mastocytosis	3	0.5
Anticonvulsants	9	1.5
Homocystinuria	2	0.3
Renal	23	4
Immobility	10	1.7
Gastro-intestinal, malabsorption and liver	41	7
Diabetes	4	0.7
Hyperparathyroidism	2	0.3
Combined (alcohol and miscellaneous)	79	13.6

Classification adapted from Allain et al., ref. 4. Numbers include other published series and personal findings.

lead to osteopenia.[9] The improvement which may occur when testosterone is prescribed for eugonadal men with spinal osteoporosis has been attributed to partial conversion of the administered hormone to oestrogen.[10]

Gonadal status is best ascertained by measuring androgen and gonadotrophic hormone blood levels. The clinical signs and symptoms of low androgen status are not reliable guides. Hypogonadism is compatible with normal-appearing genitalia and sexual function. Conversely, impotence has many causes, including diabetes, not related to low androgen status and bone mass can be normal in Klinefelter's syndrome.[11]

Alcoholism as a risk factor for osteoporosis in men has several aspects. Social drinking is associated with an increase in bone mineral density,[12] but acute inebriation results in falls. Chronic high alcohol intake leads to osteoporosis but also to falls from postural hypotension.[13] Smoking is a risk factor in young women and men by affecting the achievement of peak bone mass.[14]

ENDOCRINE CAUSES OF GENERALIZED OSTEOPOROSIS

Cushing's syndrome

Osteoporosis and spontaneous fractures were described in Cushing's original patients, and may follow prolonged treatment of patients with synthetic glucocorticoids.

Hyperthyroidism

Hyperthyroidism, either spontaneous or as a result of excessive thyroid medication, may lead to osteoporosis,[15,16] and rarely, may present as a fracture of the femoral neck.[17]

Thyrotoxicosis increases both bone accretion and bone resorption but the latter predominates. Receptors for T3 have been found in osteoblast cells in culture. There is a moderately raised serum alkaline phosphatase, indicating the increased osteoblastic activity, and increased hydroxyproline output in the urine indicating the increased osteoclastic activity. There may also be hypercalciuria. An increase in osteoid occurs when there is a very high bone turnover but, in contrast to osteomalacia, calcification rates are normal. Trabecular bone volume is also usually normal. The changes can resemble those of mild primary hyperparathyroidism and the two do sometimes coexist. The bone changes improve with treatment of the hyperthyroidism.

Mrs E was diagnosed as hypothyroid at the age of 25, and treated with thyroid extracts. At the age of 46 an attempt at withdrawal of treatment failed and since that time she received 0.1 mg of thyroxine, building up to five times per day, five days per week. At the age of 68 she presented with back pain and loss of height. X-rays showed typical osteoporotic spinal crush fractures. The serum thyroxine level was 228 mmol/l (normal: 54–142 mmol/l). The free thyroxine index was greater than 300 units (normal: 54–260 units). The thyroxine dosage was slowly reduced to 0.1 mg twice a day at which level thyroid indices became normal. Calcium equivalent to 1 g of calcium per day was given. During four years' follow-up there have been no further fractures, but she retains a typical osteoporotic stoop.

Institutionalized cretins on thyroid treatment and patients with thyroid cancer on suppressive doses of T3 are other groups at increased risk of osteoporosis, risks which may have to be accepted in balancing risks and benefits.

Hyperparathyroidism

Parathyroid hormone levels are generally raised in elderly women with osteoporosis, reflecting reduction in vitamin D activity, in turn resulting from inadequate intake or poor utilization. Supplements of vitamin D given to elderly women suppress these levels and in prospective trials have reduced the hip fracture incidence.[18,19]

Hypopituitarism

Hypopituitarism in childhood leads to impaired skeletal growth and stops sexual development. There is often osteoporosis with vertebral collapse. Hypopituitarism acquired in adult life is usually the result of haemorrhage into, or infarction of, the pituitary and in women is a rare complication of pregnancy (Sheehan's syndrome). Hypogonadism follows and with it progressive demineralization of bone.

Hyperprolactinaemia

Hyperprolactinaemia is present in 15% of women who do not ovulate. The usual cause is a pituitary adenoma. Hyperprolactinaemia leads to suppression of the pituitary–gonadal axis in both women and men causing osteoporosis unless successfully treated.[20]

Female hypogonadism

The presenting feature of hypogonadism in young women, of whatever cause, is amenorrhoea. This should always be investigated and treated. Untreated it leads to increased loss of bone mineral and fragility fractures.[21]

Anorexia nervosa and bulimia

These conditions predominantly affect young women. Young women should have at least one-fifth of their body weight as fat in order to start menstruating and slightly more to have regular cycles.[22] Body fat content less than this is associated with irregular or absent menstrual periods and low circulating oestrogen levels leading to risk of osteopenia and fracture. If the patient can be induced to eat normally and not too much time has passed the bone density which has been lost can be recovered.[23] But for those who have been severely affected for over a year or more, permanent damage to the bones will have been done.

Young female over-exercise syndrome

Up to 70% of young women endurance runners and 50% of elite professional ballet dancers experience oligomenorrhoea. Many of the dancers have a delayed menarche or do not menstruate normally until they leave the profession. The over-exercise syndrome shares with anorexia physical hyperactivity and a diet which young women believe will help them avoid putting on weight. The word 'runnerexia' has been coined to epitomize the similarities. There is less tendency than with anorexia to loss of bone density, the intense exercise exerting some protective effect[24] but not enough to overcome entirely the loss of circulating oestrogens. Reduction in bone density compared with age-matched norms is common but fracture rates are difficult to assess because of the occupational physical hazards.

Turner's syndrome

Turner's syndrome (XO) occurs in 0.5 per 1000 of live born female children. There is reduction of cortical and possibly also of trabecular bone and growth in height is reduced. Its pathogenesis may be more than simple oestrogen deficiency as osteoporosis may be apparent in affected children. Chromosome analysis confirms the diagnosis. Oestrogen treatment is necessary for pubertal sex development and to reduce the fracture risk.

Oophorectomy

Oophorectomy, whether surgical or radiological, when done before the menopause is the commonest cause of precocious female hypogonadism. It is the major indication for hormone replacement therapy. Many would think that it is unethical, and perhaps open to litigation, for a woman to be subjected to oophorectomy without being advised about and offered HRT. Yet Spector[25] found that only one-quarter of women at high risk of later osteoporosis because of hysterectomy, with or without oophorectomy, were offered HRT and then only for a short and inadequate time.

Gonadotrophin-releasing hormone agonists

Gonadotrophin-releasing hormone agonists prescribed for endometriosis stop ovarian production of oestrogen and lead to loss of bone mineral.[26]

Male hypogonadism

Osteoporosis may occur in male hypogonadism, for example after orchidectomy for testicular or prostatic cancer, childhood bilateral mumps orchiitis, castration of male transvestites, treatment of prostatic cancer with gonadotrophin-releasing hormone agonists and some instances of Klinefelter's syndrome (XXY). In the latter there is increased bone resorption with low bone formation. The patients are tall with relatively long limbs, feminine distribution of fat and pubic hair, and reduction of secondary sexual characteristics. Treatment of hypogonadism is with testosterone (see page 224).

Primary adrenocortical failure (Addison's disease)

Bone density is normal in Addison's disease in men and in premenopausal women on appropriate adrenocortical hormone supplements, but may be markedly reduced in postmenopausal women despite these supplements.[27]

Diabetes

Osteoporosis, in particular cortical osteoporosis, has been reported in diabetes, and it has been postulated that insulin deficiency may affect the protein matrix of bone. However, a large cohort study in Rochester, Minnesota,[28] failed to show any increase of fracture rate. Regional osteoporosis is common in the neuropathic diabetic foot. Generalized osteoporosis, when it occurs, may also reflect diabetic renal disease or secondary infection.

Pregnancy

Adult idiopathic generalized osteoporosis is occasionally seen in young women during or just after pregnancy (see Figure 4.4).[29,30] It develops rapidly and can cause fracture.[31] It is rare and clearly there are physiological mechanisms that normally protect against it. It can affect first or later pregnancies, but usually does not recur if a woman who has suffered from it becomes pregnant again. The cause is unknown but a significant reduction of bone density in the mothers of sufferers has been reported. The condition needs to be differentiated from transient osteoporosis of the hip which often recurs in subsequent pregnancies (see page 101).

OSTEOPOROSIS IN CHRONIC DISEASES

Rheumatoid arthritis

The great victories of medicine in the twentieth century have involved the abolition of acute infectious diseases that are fatal in the young. However, these triumphs have saved people for the chronic diseases of adulthood and old age. All chronic diseases predispose to osteoporosis. Immobilizing chronic diseases, such as stroke and rheumatoid arthritis, are particularly liable to do so so.[32] When, in addition, the disease affects a postmenopausal woman who is treated with glucocorticoids,

Table 4.2 Risk factors of osteoporosis and fracture in rheumatoid arthritis

- Postmenopausal women predominate
- Loss of mobility—local and generalized
- Glucocorticoid treatment
- Chronic inflammation and circulating mediators of bone resorption—IL-1, PGE_2
- Nutritional deficiencies
- Abnormal stressing of bones
- Falls due to locomotor instability

the risk of osteoporosis and fracture becomes very high and is attributable to a number of factors (see Table 4.2).

A low bone density early in the disease signals a poor prognosis.[33] There is an increase of radioisotope uptake by bone, not only in rheumatoid joints, but also at sites distant from affected joints. Synovitis and the erosion of subchondral bone are mediated by local factors, such as the cytokines interleukin-1 (IL-1) and prostaglandin-E_2 (PGE_2), which stimulate bone resorption and have a systemic effect (see page 18). Such cytokines are also released in other inflammatory conditions.

Early disease is mainly associated with periarticular loss of bone mass, but patients with rheumatoid arthritis treated with nonsteroidal anti-inflammatory agents alone have a low total body calcium as assessed by neutron activation analysis and dual energy X-ray absorptiometry. Active synovitis is associated with this periarticular and generalized osteoporosis. Bone mass is even lower in those who are treated with glucocorticoids.[34] Patients with rheumatoid disease, like other elderly disabled persons, are at additional risk of osteomalacia, particularly the more elderly patients who have difficulty getting outside into the sunlight and in whom depression and reduced mobility may interfere with preparing and eating a reasonable diet.

There is an increased risk of fracture, not only at conventional sites such as the neck of the femur, but of stress fracture occurring at unusual sites because of joint deformity affecting the loading of bones (see Figure 4.5). The

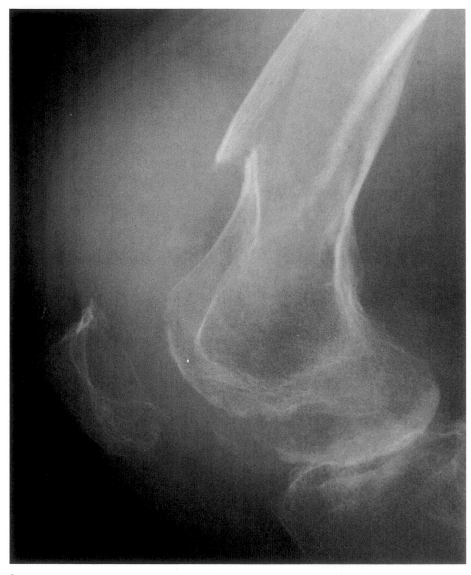

a

Figure 4.5
Stress fractures in patients with rheumatoid arthritis of (a) distal
femur, (b) several sites in the tibia and fibula, (c) the ankle
mortice and (d) the proximal fibula in a patient with knee
involvement and valgus deformity (e). These result from the
abnormal stress due to joint deformities and the increased
fragility of the bone due to immobility, inflammation and often
the use of glucocorticoids. Stress fractures in the distal lower
limb often present with the sudden onset of calf pain and may be
confused with deep vein thrombosis or a ruptured Baker's cyst.

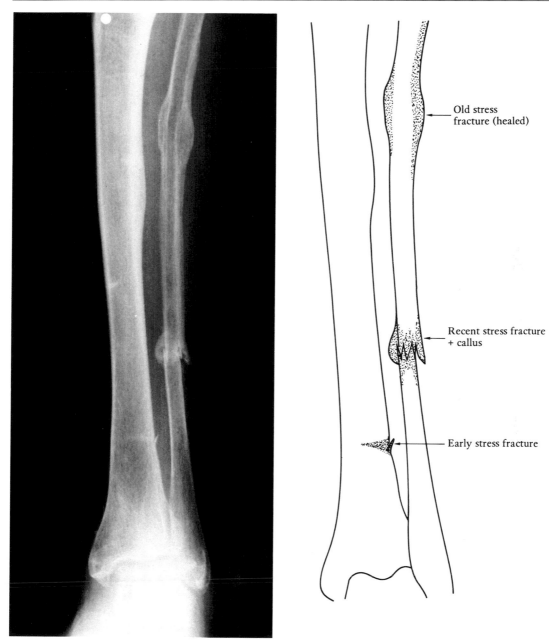

Old stress fracture (healed)

Recent stress fracture + callus

Early stress fracture

b

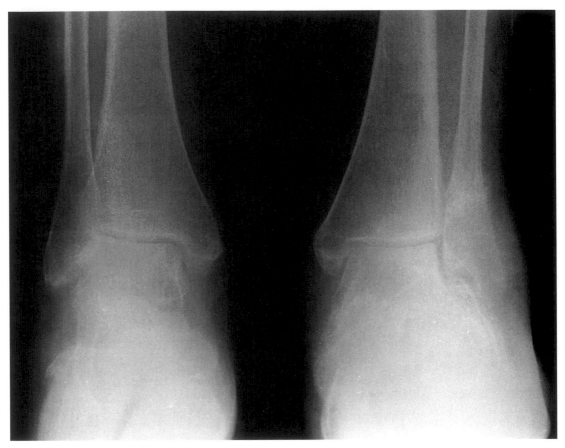

c

Figure 4.5 *continued*

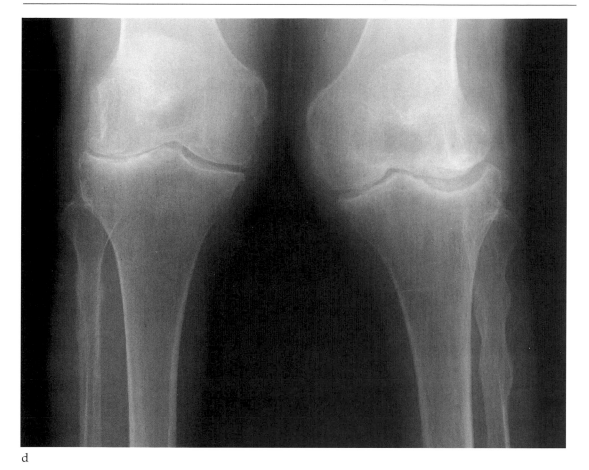

d

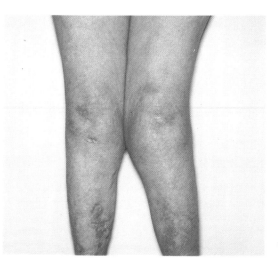

e

increased risk of fracture is about twofold and its effect can be devastating in somebody already incapacitated by joint disease.

Prevention and treatment

Prevention entails controlling synovitis, maintaining mobility and the avoidance of systemic glucocorticoids. Where these cannot be avoided deflazacort, which is more 'bone-friendly', should be considered. Major advances are better disease-modifying therapies and intra-articular therapy with long-acting forms of glucocorticoids, such as methylprednisolone acetate or triamcinolone acetonide. These can be given in relatively small doses into one or two actively inflamed joints. Where one knee is inflamed and painful, a single injection of 20 mg of triamcinolone hexacetonide may allow the patient to walk in a relatively pain-free manner and thus remain mobile when, but for such an injection, he or she would have been confined to a bed-and-chair existence.

Ankylosing spondylitis

The predisposing factors for osteoporosis in rheumatoid arthritis apply also to ankylosing spondylitis. In this disease loss of bone density in the spine can precede detectable radiological changes. In late disease the rigid spine is osteoporotic and brittle. Fractures through the spine are not uncommon and are very painful as the fracture line may be the only point in the spine where movement is possible. Fracture of a rigid neck in ankylosing spondylitis is one of the few ways in which this disease can directly cause death. Prevention of loss of bone density relies on regular and vigorous exercise and when necessary anti-osteoporosis drugs, particularly one of the bisphosphonates. Measurement of bone density is recommended to determine when it is necessary to intervene.

Other inflammatory rheumatic diseases

Osteopenia is common in the seronegative arthropathies, in systemic sclerosis, systemic lupus erythematosus and polymyalgia rheumatica.

Alimentary system disorders and generalized osteoporosis

Chronic liver diseases

All forms of chronic liver diseases may be associated with osteoporosis. This tendency is most marked in primary biliary cirrhosis where osteoporosis is almost inevitable. Osteoporosis has also been reported in 25–50% of patients with haemochromatosis, chronic active hepatitis, chronic alcoholic liver disease and chronic cholestatic jaundice. An increasing number of patients with liver disease are now being treated with liver transplantation. They require the use of long-term glucocorticoids and immunosuppressives which predispose to skeletal failure. Osteomalacia, of mild degree, is also often associated with liver disease, appearing together with the osteoporosis.

Calcium deficiency in chronic liver disease occurs for a number of reasons. Insufficient vitamin D may result from chronic ill health and lack of UV light, from malabsorption due to deficient bile salts, or from impairment of hepatic 25-hydroxylase and the failure to convert vitamin D to active metabolites. There may be a poor dietary intake of calcium or that which is taken may be bypassed bound to undigested fats and thus poorly absorbed. Glucocorticoids, either endogenous (raised in liver disease), or exogenous due to treatment, impair calcium absorption. There are factors that predispose also to osteomalacia, but vitamin D does not correct all the osteopenia found in primary biliary cirrhosis.

Malabsorption syndromes

All chronic causes of alimentary malabsorption are associated with osteoporosis and osteomalacia of variable degree. Gluten sensitivity (coeliac disease), postgastrectomy and blind loop syndromes are perhaps the commonest.

Treatment

Calcium supplements have been shown to prevent loss of bone mass in liver disease and even to increase bone cortical width on the metacarpal index (see page 216). Calcium absorption improves in malabsorption if the underlying cause can be cured, for example by a gluten-free diet in coeliac disease or by appropriate antibiotics or surgery in blind loop syndromes, Crohn's or Whipple's diseases. Slow release magnesium chloride preparations and vitamin D supplements should also be given.

Osteoporosis in chronic lung disease

Osteoporosis occurs in chronic obstructive airways disease and chronic asthma treated with glucocorticoids. Respiratory acidosis may

be a further factor. Vertebral collapse may be difficult to treat as any effective spinal support further restricts breathing.

Neurological disease and generalized osteoporosis

Immobility, depending on its extent, rapidly leads to generalized or localized osteoporosis.

In *paraplegia*, the degree of osteoporosis depends on the level of the spinal cord damage and on the daily care and treatment that the paraplegic receives. The loss of the use of the legs is often compensated for by great increases in the power of the arms. This allows younger paraplegics, with suitable training and if necessary braces, to walk with crutches, or an implantable neurological device encouraging some degree of automatic activity in the muscles of the legs, which helps slow down the otherwise inevitable osteoporosis. Careful

---

Mrs J E was a thin, rather wasted 51-year-old woman suffering from asthma and widespread chronic atopic eczema, which had been treated with glucocorticoid ointments and tablets. Spinal osteoporosis developed and glucocorticoid treatment was reduced, but it was not possible to reduce the dose to below 2.5 mg of prednisolone per day. Cyclical oestrogen/progestogen treatment and calcium supplements were given to protect against further osteoporosis.

Mrs E V had suffered from multiple sclerosis for 23 years and had been confined to a wheelchair for the previous 13 years. She was admitted to hospital with a diagnosis of left-sided deep leg vein thrombosis. She had a bed sore on the sacrum and had been looked after devotedly at home by her husband. The referring general practitioner described the leg as 'classically large, white and oedematous', but it was noted that there was no tenderness in the calf. The admitting doctor concurred with the diagnosis at first and started anticoagulant treatment. Bruising became apparent and an X-ray disclosed a spiral fracture of the upper third of the left femur and extreme osteoporosis (see Figure 4.6). There was a history of a mid-shaft fracture of the left tibia after minor trauma one year previously. The patient's husband subsequently attempted to sue the hospital for causing the fracture, but was dissuaded by his advisers.

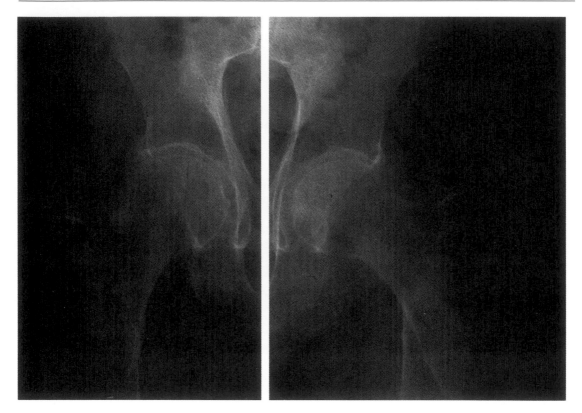

Figure 4.6
A painless spiral fracture of the upper third of the left femur in a 58-year-old woman immobilized for 13 years by multiple sclerosis.

nursing and training will enable patients to avoid pressure sores and ulcers of skin deprived of sensory input, sores which otherwise become chronically infected, contributing to local osteoporosis. Immobility in the paraplegic is to be discouraged if at all possible. Wheelchair sports of all kinds and avoidance of the all too common obesity are among the measures that should receive attention.

In patients with *progressive multiple sclerosis*, the gradual loss of mobility leads to a bedfast state when osteoporosis is inevitable. Osteoporotic fractures of long bones may occur just in lifting the patient, to the embar-

rassment and distress of caring relatives and nurses.[35]

Muscular dystrophies, when advanced, are usually complicated by disuse osteoporosis. *Anterior poliomyelitis*, fortunately now rare, in its more disabling forms was associated with generalized and localized osteoporosis.

Skin diseases

Several skin diseases require long-term glucocorticoid therapy which can result in osteoporosis. Severe chronic exfoliative dermatitis of the 'homme rouge' type, with its failure of normal integumentary control of heat and evaporation losses and general immobilization, is followed by osteoporosis. Similar effects are seen in chronic severe exfoliative psoriasis, pemphigus and mycosis fungoides. These conditions are, also, usually complicated by the osteoporotic effects of concurrent corticosteroid treatment.

In urticaria pigmentosa (mastocytosis), osteoporosis may lead to spinal crush fractures. Sometimes the mastocytosis and osteoporosis precede the typical rash.[36]

REGIONAL OSTEOPOROSIS

Disuse

Disuse of a limb produces a rapid loss of bone mass from that limb, irrespective of whether the disuse is attributable to immobilization after a fracture or to pain, joint disease or paralysis. More widespread osteoporosis occurs after prolonged immobilization of the whole patient by coma or stroke, but even after stroke it is the bones of the paretic limb that are most affected. Simple bed-rest without any underlying disease also leads to loss of bone. In experimental animals, immobilization of a limb by paralysis or by encasing in a plaster of Paris cast leads to regional osteoporosis, while in man the weightlessness of space flight has provided a model for studying disuse bone loss.

Conversely, bone mass is increased with locally increased muscular activity, such as hypertrophy of the metatarsal bones in ballet dancers or of the bones of the dominant arm in professional tennis players. Moreover, local bone mass lost during immobilization can largely be restored by remobilization and progressive exercising.

Thus, bone, a living structure which is continuously being formed and broken down,

settles at a dynamic equilibrium where the bone is strong enough for the demands upon it. The messages that bones receive and which enable them to respond to the degree of use are not yet fully known. It is clear, however, that bones need constant feedback signals from the stresses which muscles exert at their attachments to bone and from the transmitted loads of body weight and of acceleration during movement. The normal development of bone in children also depends on maintained functional activity.

Immobility bone loss

The increase in bone loss with immobility is the result of an up to threefold increase in bone resorption which can occur in the first few weeks and is reflected by a rapid increase in urinary calcium and hydroxyproline excretion. This is only partly compensated for by a small increase in local bone formation. A small rise in plasma calcium may also be detected but hypercalcaemia is rare and is normally only seen with severe immobilization such as following a high paraplegia. It has been postulated that the rise in blood calcium suppresses plasma parathyroid hormone (PTH) and vitamin D levels and these, in turn, cause a decrease in calcium absorption. The hypercalciuria of immobilization may predispose to renal calculus formation in paraplegics. The rate of local resorption gradually decreases in those patients whose immobility persists until a new equilibrium at a lower level is reached after one to two years. By this time up to 40% of trabecular bone will have been lost.

Bone loss is more rapid in weight-bearing bones than in nonweight-bearing bones and more in trabecular bone than in cortical bone. Radiologically apparent osteoporosis develops within two to three months, sooner in younger persons or where there has been more extensive immobilization. When mobility is restored bone density increases, although this process is much slower and sometimes incomplete.

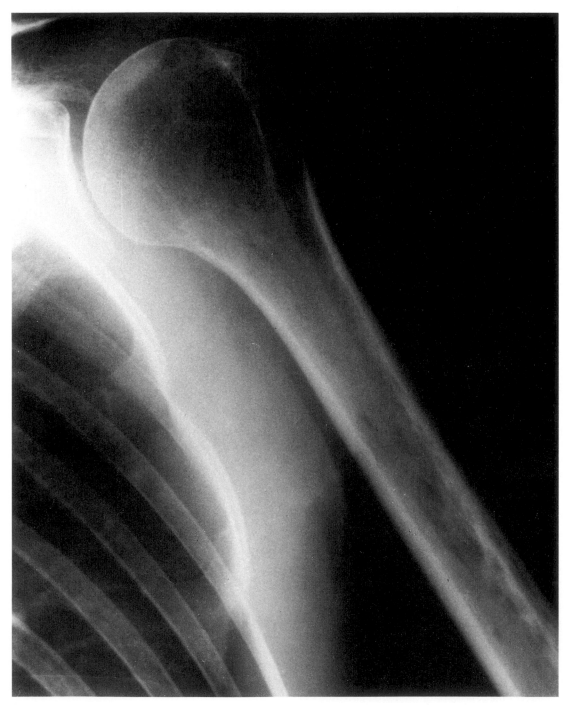

a

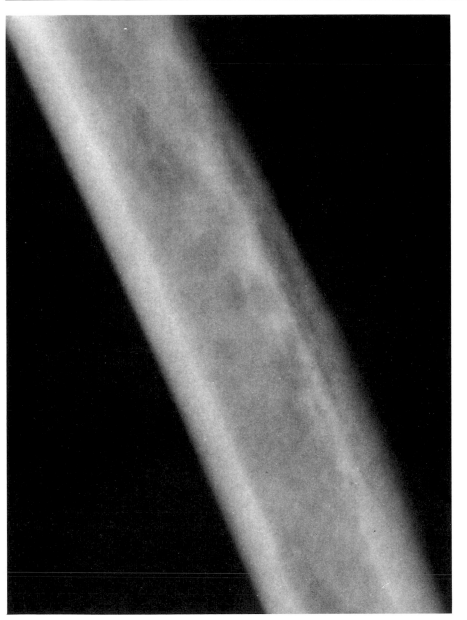

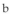
b

Figure 4.7
(a) Disuse osteoporosis of the humerus following
adhesive capsulitis of the shoulder. Relatively well
defined ellipsoid radiolucencies can be seen in the
long axis of the bone. (b) The resorption of the cortex
results in blurring of the corticomedullary junction.

There is a risk of fracture of the osteoporotic bones during this period before full restoration of bone.

Various radiological patterns of bone loss following immobility have been described (see Figure 4.7). A uniform osteopenia is common. A loss of the fine trabecular pattern without cortical thinning may occur, and is seen in carpal and tarsal bones and at the ends of the long bones. In more acute osteoporosis a speckled or spotty loss of bone occurs at similar sites. Other patterns are linear translucent bands, which may appear either as 4–8 mm bands across the entire width of the long bones, becoming less apparent as generalized osteopenia develops, or small subcortical translucent bands that can occur as an early change. A narrow translucent zone in the immediate subchondral position is often seen when immobilization is the result of acute joint disease. However, cortical changes are sometimes the only ones observed: these include subperiosteal and endosteal scalloping or lamellation, particularly seen in the shafts of the metatarsals, followed by narrowing of the cortical width as compared with the total width of the shaft. These changes are generally reversible and the cortex is the last to recover. However, if trabeculae are totally lost they cannot reappear. Bone is then deposited on the remaining trabecular structures so that fine trabeculation is replaced by coarse trabeculation, which may not confer the same amount of strength on the bone.

Treatment

With regional immobilization of one or more limbs, preventive measures must be taken as early as possible. Treatment should aim first at control of pain, and subsequently at the cause of immobilization. Thus, isometric exercises can be practised even inside a plaster immobilizing a limb. For immobilization due to paralysis, electrical stimulation of muscles can help to depress bone loss but efforts are generally directed at trying to maintain and improve the function of any residual muscle units.

Drugs, apart from those to relieve pain, have a secondary place. Anabolic steroids (such as nandrolone decanoate in oil, 25 mg by intramuscular injection) have been used. They decrease bone resorption and may be helpful in the initial high turnover phase. An increased allowance of calcium in the diet would help to counteract the increased calcium loss in the urine. Hydrochlorothiazide, 50 mg twice daily, monitored by 24-hour urinary calcium excretion measurements, has the same effect. Calcitonin and bisphosphonates are as yet unproven. Naturally, the more rapidly the period of immobilization can be overcome and the more physically active the patient can remain, the less serious will be the problem of regional osteoporosis.

Reflex sympathetic dystrophy (Sudeck's atrophy, algodystrophy)

The reflex sympathetic dystrophy syndrome has been known for more than a century. Following an initiating event, the commonest of which is local trauma (in particular a fracture, or damage to a peripheral nerve), a part of the body shows localized wasting of all tissues, accompanied by severe pain, often of a burning character. Most commonly a hand or a foot is affected but it is not unknown in other areas, including the patella. The area affected is painful and tender, and often cannot be moved. Reflex sympathetic dystrophy can be divided into three stages:

1) At first the skin is warm, shiny and oedematous and there may also be an increase in hair and nail growth and sweating. This phase may last six months.
2) A dystrophic phase then follows, lasting about three months, with the skin becoming cold, oedematous and often cyanotic. There is loss of hair, brittle nails and the limitation of joint motion persists.

3) In the final atrophic phase the skin is thin and there is atrophy of the underlying soft tissues. Pain is now often intractable and joints may become rigid, sometimes with ankylosis. Amputation may even be advisable in extreme cases.

Osteoporosis can appear radiologically as early as four to eight weeks and is obvious by the dystrophic phase. In the final phase of atrophy the fractures occur.

> A 56-year-old man developed severe angina and had a coronary artery bypass graft. Postoperative cardiac output was poor and a balloon pump was inserted via the right femoral artery. The patient subsequently made a good recovery but complained of pain in his right leg, which was initially attributed to the femoral artery cannulation. However, his symptoms became severe and it was clear that the pain was located in the patella, which was warm and tender, with overlying skin discoloration. The X-ray showed rapidly progressive osteopenia of the patella and the radioisotope bone scan showed an increased uptake (see Figure 4.8). A diagnosis of reflex sympathetic dystrophy was made. Symptoms have shown little response to any treatment.

The osteoporosis may be dramatic (see case history above and Figures 4.8 and 4.9), and disuse is probably an important contributing factor to its rapidity. Radiologically, it develops a typical speckled or spotty ground glass appearance. The bone loss may be such that on X-ray there may even appear to be erosions of subchondral bone. Radioisotope bone scanning is positive, and may be bilateral despite unilateral signs and symptoms. Where this syndrome occurs near a joint it may masquerade as an acute monarthritis and the possibility of sepsis is often raised. On examination, however, the pain is found to be in the periarticular structures.

The pathogenesis is unknown, but a trigger is required. It is associated with increased activity of the sympathetic nervous system.

Treatment

Treatment involves adequate analgesia to control pain and then progressive and persistent attempts at mobilization and restoration of function (often best carried out in the hydrotherapy pool). Sympathetic blockade, either of the sympathetic chain or by means of intravenous regional sympathetic blocks with guanethidine, is sometimes effective in the early stages. Transcutaneous nerve stimulation may help relieve pain. In many patients it may take up to 18 months before recovery, but a minority never recover, the affected part becoming increasingly useless and atrophic. Various bisphosphonates have been given, usually by the intravenous route, and rapid relief of pain reported, with later improvement in limb function and bone density.[37]

Transient regional osteoporosis

Allied to reflex sympathetic dystrophy, but not so severe, is transient regional osteoporosis, a self-limiting condition lasting up to one year in any one site, characterized by pain and disability, and with rapidly developing osteoporosis in the subjacent bone. There is usually no obvious initiating factor and it is reversible. Two well recognized patterns occur.

Transient osteoporosis of the hip

Transient osteoporosis of the hip affects children and young to middle-aged adults, mainly females. In women, typically the left hip is affected in the third trimester of pregnancy. In men, either hip can be involved. Patients present with hip pain which is sometimes

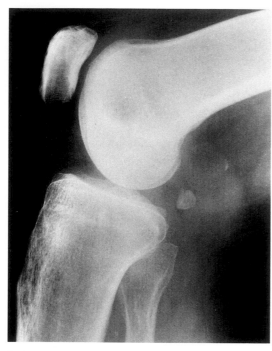

a

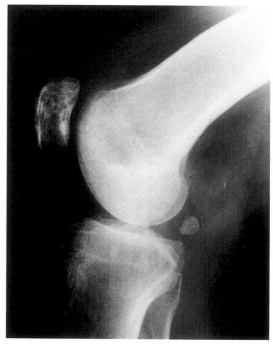

b

Figure 4.8
(a, b) X-rays of right knee two months apart showing rapidly progressive osteoporosis of the patella and tibia. (c) The radioisotope bone scan shows increased uptake.

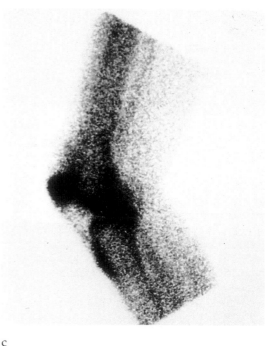

referred to the anterior knee on weight-bearing. The erythrocyte sedimentation rate or plasma viscosity are occasionally elevated but this may be difficult to interpret in pregnant women. There may be an effusion but synovial biopsies have only occasionally shown mild chronic inflammatory changes. Complete recovery in two to six months is the rule.

Radioisotope bone scans can be positive before radiological changes. The X-rays show marked demineralization of the femoral head and to a lesser extent of the femoral neck and acetabulum (see Figure 4.10). The joint space, that is the thickness of the cartilage, remains normal.

c

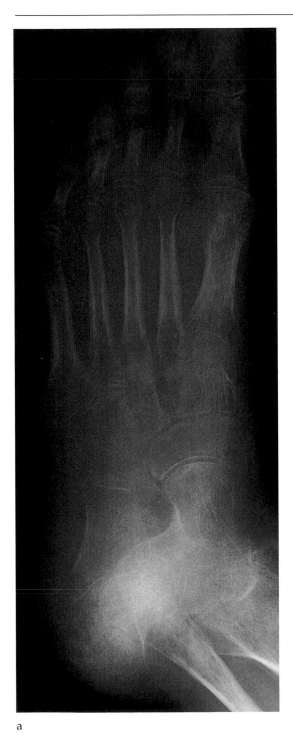

a

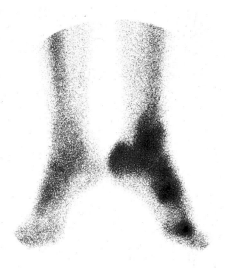

b

Figure 4.9
Reflex sympathetic dystrophy more typically affects the distal limbs. The X-ray (a) of this foot shows marked osteoporosis and the radioisotope bone scan (b) shows increased uptake.

Regional migratory osteoporosis

Regional migratory osteoporosis is similar but more commonly affects the knee, ankle and foot. There is pain, swelling, oedema and often muscle atrophy followed by rapidly developing osteoporosis. It heals in one site only to recur elsewhere. Typically two to four attacks occur over three years, but durations of up to 13 years have been reported. Recovery between episodes may be complete.

Radioisotope bone scans are positive for the affected areas. X-ray of the affected areas shows rapidly developing diffuse and patchy demineralization with cortical thinning and occasionally a periosteal reaction. These changes resolve within two years, although some loss of trabecular bone may persist.

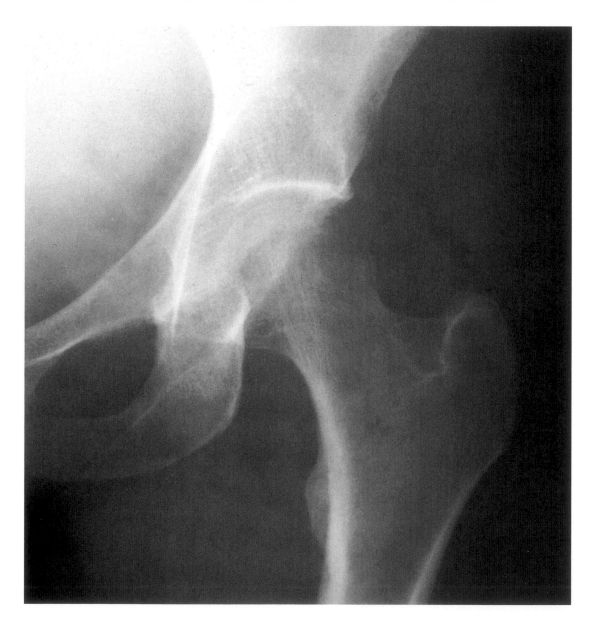

Figure 4.10
Transient osteoporosis of the hip in a 29-year-old
woman who developed a painful hip during
pregnancy. The radiograph shows marked
osteoporosis; the patient eventually recovered
postpartum.

The differential diagnosis includes an acute monarthritis, local sepsis, granulomatous and neoplastic conditions and the localized acute osteoporotic phase of Paget's disease.

DRUGS AND OTHER RISK FACTORS

Glucocorticoids

Osteoporosis was described in 1932 in Cushing's original patients with excess endogenous glucocorticoid secretion and was soon recognized as a complication of the use of glucocorticoids and adrenocorticotrophic hormone after their introduction in the late 1940s. The extent of loss of bone mass reflects both the dose and duration of treatment. Instances of fracture have, however, been reported to occur spontaneously within weeks of commencing glucocorticoid treatment. Trabecular bone is preferentially affected, especially in the vertebral bodies and ribs.

A 53-year-old man (see Figure 4.11) developed a mononeuritis multiplex with bilateral wrist drop and loss of sensation over the right foot, associated with loss of weight, and pain and swelling of his knees. The diagnosis of polyarteritis nodosa was confirmed by angiography and he responded to treatment with 40 mg of prednisolone per day. However, he became diabetic and hypertensive. Cyclophosphamide was introduced as a steroid-sparing agent but he became neutropenic and septicaemic. He was therefore continued on the lowest dose of prednisolone, between 12.5 mg and 20 mg per day, to control disease activity. After nine months he complained of low back pain and it was observed that he had lost height and developed a kyphosis. X-ray confirmed spinal osteoporosis with wedging and loss of height of several thoracic vertebrae. He also noted thinning of the skin and easy bruising.

Crush fractures of the tibial tables may lead to valgus or varus deformity.

A 70-year-old woman (see Figure 4.12) developed painful knees and had been treated with prednisolone 10 mg per day during the previous three years. She suddenly developed severe pain in the left knee and the X-ray showed a medial tibial plateau fracture and osteoarthritis. The isotope scan showed the fracture and also the bone reaction in the joint associated with the osteoarthritis. There was no evidence of an inflammatory arthritis and steroids were discontinued.

The effect of glucocorticoids is additional to the other osteoporosis risk factors, i.e., being elderly, immobile or postmenopausal. Children with juvenile chronic arthritis or severe asthma treated with glucocorticoids are also at risk and show an increased incidence of vertebral fractures. Men are at risk but less so. High dose glucocorticoids, even when given only as short courses, either as intravenous or oral prednisolone, may also be associated with

A three-year-old boy presented with fever, rash and joint pains and the diagnosis of systemic juvenile chronic arthritis was made. He was initially treated with aspirin, but after 10 months of active disease, he developed pericarditis and glucocorticoids were commenced. It was difficult to reduce prednisolone below 15 mg per day without a flare in rash, fever and arthritis so severe that he was confined to his bed. Whilst on prednisolone he gained 3 kg in weight over four months, became very 'cushingoid' in his face and lost some height. Radiological examination showed osteoporotic collapse of vertebral bodies.

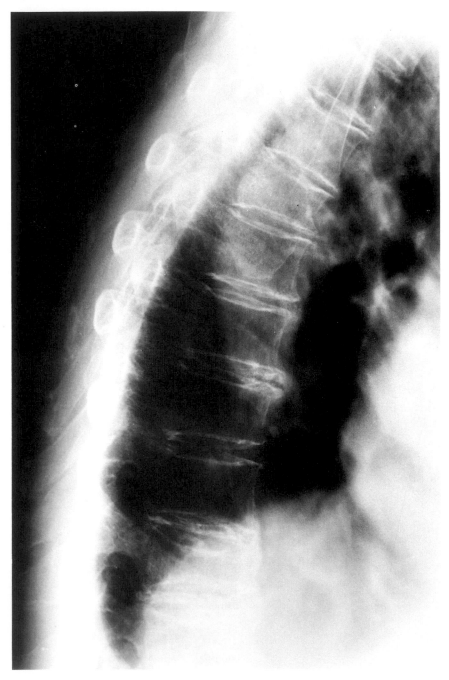

Figure 4.11
Osteoporosis of the thoracic spine with a wedge
fracture associated with glucocorticoid therapy.

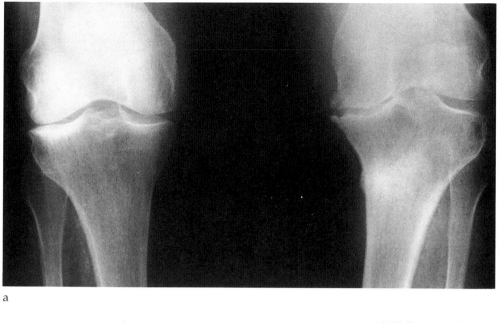

a

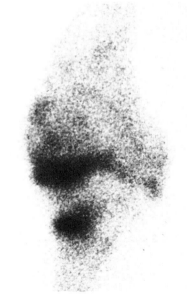

b

Figure 4.12
(a) Medial tibial plateau fracture of the left knee in a woman inappropriately treated with glucocorticoids for osteoarthritis of the knee. (b) Radioisotope bone scan showing increased uptake associated with fracture and osteoarthritis.

an increased risk of avascular necrosis, in particular of the femoral head. Glucocorticoids may retard growth in the immature skeleton, but this is less marked with alternate day therapy.

Glucocorticoid treatment decreases bone formation and increases bone resorption. The decreased formation is most evident in trabecular bone. There is a direct effect on osteoblasts, with reduction of the recruitment of progenitor cells and the synthesis of bone matrix. There is a small increase in the number of osteoclasts and resorbing surfaces. Glucocorticoids also reduce intestinal calcium absorption and increase urinary calcium excretion. In some patients there is a small increase in circulating immunoreactive PTH. In animals, parathyroidectomy abolishes the glucocorticoid-mediated increase in bone resorption. In addition, glucocorticoids suppress the adrenal production of precursor steroids which are the main source, when metabolized, of oestrogen in postmenopausal women. Glucocorticoids have an important catabolic and proteolytic activity, which is particularly marked in skin collagen. Skin becomes thin, atrophic and typical glucocorticoid bruises become apparent as the supporting tissue for the capillaries is weakened. A similar damaging effect no doubt occurs in bone collagen. The synthetic glucocorticoid deflazacort is more 'bone friendly' than prednisolone at an equal anti-inflammatory dose: 6 mg of deflazacort has about the same anti-inflammatory effect as 5 mg of prednisolone.[38]

Management

It is a counsel of perfection to avoid glucocorticoid treatment altogether. In many diseases there is no substitute. The dose must be continuously monitored and kept to a minimum. There is no safe daily dose as there appears to be considerable variation between individual patients in their resistance to the osteopenic effect of glucocorticoids. In general, the dose should be kept at the equivalent of 7.5 mg per day of prednisolone, less if possible. Total dose given is also important and treatment should be for as short a period as is practicable. The use of the 1 mg-size tablets of prednisolone allows small weekly decrements of dosage. In children, but not in adults, there is evidence that alternate day treatment is less damaging.

It is possible that in some conditions, such as polymyalgia rheumatica, the relatively small dose of corticosteroid needed to keep the patient comfortable and free from immobilizing stiffness is balanced in its bone-damaging effect by the greater pain-free physical activity which the patient can undertake. In diseases requiring higher doses, the possibility of using a glucocorticoid-sparing agent such as azathioprine should be considered. This has been shown to be effective in rheumatoid arthritis and in polymyalgia rheumatica.

Not all patients treated with glucocorticoids develop osteoporosis. Those most at risk can be identified by the presence of multiple predisposing factors or by measurement of bone density by absorptiometry. The disease being treated with glucocorticoids may also predispose to osteoporosis, as well as the age and menopausal status if a woman. Bone density is the best predictor of risk of future fracture and it is good practice to measure bone density of the hips and lumbar spine before starting a patient on glucocorticoid treatment, i.e., where the dose exceeds 7.5 mg a day of prednisolone or equivalent, or where the treatment is expected to be taken over at least six months or intermittently for six months in a year. If the bone mineral density T score is more than 2.5 standard deviations below the young adult mean then treatment to prevent bone loss is recommended.

The risk of serious osteoporosis on high dose or long-term glucocorticoid treatment should be explained beforehand. Where this has not been done, and osteoporotic fractures have supervened, doctors have been sued for negligence.

All patients on glucocorticoid treatment, even on small doses, should take the general lifestyle measures: have an adequate calcium and vitamin D intake (see Chapter 9), take regular weight-bearing exercise if the illness being treated permits, stop smoking, keep alcohol intake below 21 units per week (men) or 14 units (women) and try to get at least three to four hours a week exposure of the skin to sun in the summer.

For those at greatest risk, either due to high-dose and long duration of glucocorticoid treatment, the presence of other risk factors or a low bone density, the use of deflazacort should be considered. Hormone replacement therapy is effective in stopping bone loss in postmenopausal women taking glucocorticoids,[39] and should be recommended for as long as glucocorticoid treatment continues and preferably for 10 years after that to retard postmenopausal bone loss (see Chapter 8). For men, and for women for whom HRT is unsuitable, bisphosphonates are the next choice. The bisphosphonate etidronate given cyclically reduces bone loss in glucocorticoid-treated patients.[40] Calcitonins are effective, but seldom more so than bisphosphonates and are expensive for long-term use.

Fractures in glucocorticoid-treated patients

When a fracture is shown by X-ray, other diagnoses should be excluded by a full blood count, measurements of thyroid liver and renal function. For men who have fractured check the serum testosterone level and if low, consider testosterone treatment.

Heparin and oral anticoagulants

There have been several case reports of generalized osteoporosis and spontaneous fractures occurring in patients treated with more than 15 000 units of heparin daily for more than six months[41] on anticoagulant programmes. It is rare, as in a series of more than 100 patients treated with 10 000 units or less of heparin daily for up to 15 years, no such complications were seen.

Low molecular weight heparin is less toxic to the bones than standard heparin. Osteoporosis and spinal fractures in patients treated with heparin during pregnancy to prevent placental thromboses associated with recurrent miscarriage have been reported. However, idiopathic osteoporosis has not necessarily been excluded. Mast cells which secrete heparin also secrete histamine, prostaglandins, leukotrienes, 5-hydroxy-tryptamine and neutral proteases. Systemic mastocytosis is associated with osteolytic lesions rather than osteoporosis. Most indications for heparin treatment require only short-term exposure of the patient and osteoporosis is not really a danger. Long-term use of oral anticoagulants is also associated with reduced bone density.[42]

Gonadotropin releasing hormone (GnRH) agonists

GnRH agonists, which are more slowly metabolized than naturally occurring GnRH, inhibit the release of follicle-stimulating and luteinizing hormones. Thus, oestrogen production by the ovary is inhibited. This may relieve the pain of endometriosis, but there is a price to pay, including menopausal symptoms and demineralization of bones.[43]

Long-acting progesterone preparations

Depo-Provera (Upjohn, Crawley, Sussex) and Norplant (Roussel, Denham) are long-acting preparations of the progestogens medroxyprogesterone acetate and levonorgestrel, respectively. They are used as contraceptives and have variable effects on bone density.

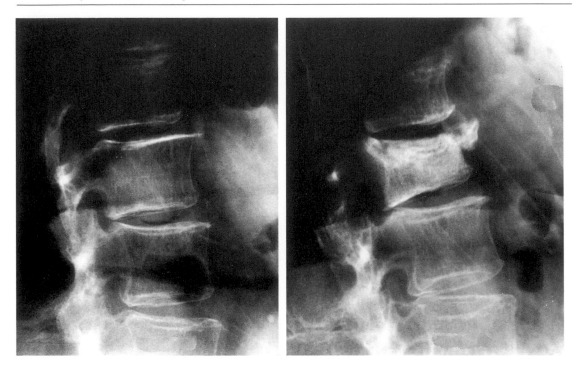

Figure 4.13
Alcoholism, osteoporosis and multiple intervertebral disc degeneration. A 70-year-old female alcoholic complained of the sudden onset of lumbar pain with referral to inguinal region and thighs. X-rays show recent crush fracture of the third lumbar vertebra with callus formation. The gas shadows in the adjacent discs can just be made out.

Early use probably increases bone density but prolonged use is associated with suppression of oestrogen formation with reduction in bone density. Bone density may recover on stopping the drugs.[44]

Alcohol

Bone mass is reduced in alcoholism with increased resorption of bone and an increased risk of fracture. This may be explained by liver disease, poor diet, lack of exposure to sunlight, and alcohol-induced calcium diuresis—the combination of factors varying for individual patients. There is also an increased risk of falls leading to fracture. In Lalor et al.'s series of 22 patients with chronic alcohol abuse,[45] none had clinical evidence of metabolic bone disease but on bone biopsy six had osteoporosis, three had osteomalacia and two had both conditions combined. The presence of osteoporosis was related to the severity of concurrent liver disease and was most advanced in those who drank only spirits (see Figure 4.13). In contrast, modest use of alcohol has been associated with protection against osteoporosis.[46]

Smoking

Premenopausal women who smoke have a tendency in later life to develop osteoporosis associated with reduced body fat and impairment of conversion by fatty tissue of precursor steroids to oestrogens. Smoking has been associated with earlier menopause and even 'passive smokers', women who live with heavy smokers but do not smoke themselves, show the effect in earlier menopause.[47] There is some dispute as to whether the effect of smoking is entirely related to coincidental slim body build, with loss of the contribution of body fat to the total oestrogen experience. The effect in advancing the age of the menopause would suggest more basic mechanisms in the association of osteoporosis and smoking. Older men who smoke do not show unexpected loss of bone density,[48] even though this tendency has been shown in young adult men.[14]

Dietary salt

A 100 mg daily salt supplement in postmenopausal women increased their daily net calcium loss from about 1 mmol/day by a further 0.57 mmol/day.[49] Consider ways of reducing dietary salt and using potassium-rich salt substitutes.

Lactose intolerance

The majority of people in the world lose the ability to digest lactose as they grow out of childhood. For them, the ingestion of lactose may cause distension and diarrhoea, and make them averse to dairy products. The capacity to digest lactose as adults is maintained in certain populations, mainly those of northern European descent; thus in Birmingham, England 3% of white people, 55% of Indian origin and 82% of Afrocaribbeans had lactase deficiency.[50] These proportions may alter with age as 60% of white New Zealand women over 60 years old were lactase-deficient compared with 12% of young women.[51] Deficiency of the enzyme is seldom absolute. Lactose intolerance is associated with intestinal hurry and impaired calcium absorption. A yeast-derived enzyme is available which can be added to milk overnight to split lactose into glucose and galactose.

Other clinical associations of osteoporosis

There is increasing evidence that the association between loss of bone density with ageing and loss of teeth because of alveolar ridge retraction may be in part causal.[52,53]

Other conditions where an increased liability to osteoporosis and fragility fractures have been reported include: severe haemophilia A; mild osteogenesis imperfecta after the menopause and homocysteinaemia in elderly women; complete androgen insensitivity (testicular feminization syndrome); and galactosaemia associated with ovarian failure. But there are many other causes.[54–58]

PRACTICAL POINTS

- Generalized osteoporosis can be divided into that mainly affecting cortical bone or trabecular bone.

- Cortical bone failure usually involves long bone fracture, which heals normally.

- Bone structural failure in the spine (mainly trabecular bone) results in wedging or crushing of vertebral bodies, with progressive and irreversible spinal shrinkage, frequent deformity and associated complications.

- Long bone fractures are usually preceded by a fall and are painful. Fractures of vertebral bodies may occur spontaneously, sometimes without pain.

- Exercise increases bone mass and immobilization leads to bone loss via increased resorption.

- Osteoporosis can be localized as in reflex sympathetic dystrophy and transient regional osteoporosis.

- Chronic disorders, such as rheumatoid arthritis, liver disease, lung disease, neurological disorders and endocrinal disorders predispose to osteoporosis.

- Osteoporosis is associated with the use of various drugs, particularly glucocorticoids.

REFERENCES

1. Smith R. Idiopathic osteoporosis in the young. *J Bone Joint Surg* (1980), **62B**: 417–27.
2. Bordier PJ, Miravet L, Hioco D. Young adult osteoporosis. *Clin Endocrinol Metab* (1973), **2**: 277–92.
3. Jackson WPU. Osteoporosis of unknown cause in younger people. *J Bone Joint Surg* (1958), **40B**: 420–41.
4. Allain T, Pitt P, Moniz C. Osteoporosis in men. *Br Med J* (1992), **305**: 955–6.
5. Devogelaer JP, Vanden Berrghe M, Nagent de Deuxchaisnes C. Osteoporosis in males is chiefly a secondary condition. *Bone* (1995), **16** (suppl 1): 1855.
6. Ringe JD, Dorst A. Osteoporosis in males, pathogenesis and clinical classification. *Proceedings of the Fourth International Symposium on Osteoporosis and Consensus Development Conference*, Hong Kong, 27 March–2 April 1993. Rødovre: Denmark (1993), p. 184.
7. Anderson FH, Francis RM. Androgen supplementation in eugonadal men with osteoporosis: effects of six months' treatment on bone mineral density and cardiovascular risk factors. *Bone* (1995), **16** (suppl 1): 159.
8. Stanley HL, Schmitt BP, Poses RM et al. Does hypogonadism contribute to the occurrence of minimal trauma hip fracture in elderly men? *J Am Geriatr Soc* (1991), **39**: 766–71.
9. Finkelstein JS, Meer RM, Biller BM et al. Osteoporosis in men with a history of delayed puberty. *N Engl J Med* (1992), **326**: 600–4.
10. Anderson F, Francis R, Hindmarsch P et al. Serum oestradiol in osteoporotic and normal men is related to bone mineral density. *Osteoporos Int* (1996), **6** (suppl 1): 60.
11. Luisetto G, Mastrogiacomo I, Bonani G et al. Bone mass and mineral metabolism in Klinefelter's syndrome. *Osteoporos Int* (1995), **5**: 455–61.
12. Holbrook TL, Barret-Connor E. A prospective study of alcohol and bone mineral density. *Br Med J* (1993), **306**: 1506–9.
13. Burke V, Beilin LJ, Geran R et al. Postural fall in blood pressure in the elderly in relation to drug treatment and other life style factors. *Q J Med* (1992), **84**: 583–91.

14. Valimaki MJ, Karkkainen M, Lamberg-Allardt C et al. Exercise, smoking and calcium intake during adolescence and early adulthood as determinants of peak bone mass. *Br Med J* (1994), **309**: 230–5.

15. Schneider DL, Barrett-Connor E, Morton DJ. Thyroid hormone use and bone mineral density in elderly women: effects of estrogen. *JAMA* (1994), **271**: 1245–9.

16. Franklyn JA, Betteridge J, Daykin J et al. Long-term thyroxine treatment and bone mineral density. *Lancet* (1992), **340**: 9–13.

17. Francis RM, Barnett MJ, Selby P et al. Thyrotoxicosis presenting as a fracture of the femoral neck. *Br Med J* (1982), **285**: 97–8.

18. Chapuy MC, Arlot ME, Duboeuf F et al. Vitamin D_3 to prevent hip fractures in elderly women. *N Engl J Med* (1992), **327**: 1673–82.

19 Heikinheimo RJ, Incovaara JA, Harju EJ et al. Annual injection of Vitamin D and fractures of aged bones. *Calcif Tissue Int* (1992), **51**: 105–10.

20. Management of prolactinoma [Editorial]. *Lancet* (1990), **336**: 661.

21. Davies MC, Hall ML, Jacobs HS. Bone mineral loss in young women with amenorrhoea. *Br Med J* (1990), **301**: 790–3.

22. Frisch RE. Fatness, menarche and female fertility. *Perspect Biol Med* (1985), **28**: 611–33.

23. Treasure JI, Russell GFM, Fogelman I et al. Reversible bone loss in anorexia nervosa. *Br Med J* (1987), **295**: 474–5.

24. Wolman RL, Clark P, McNally E et al. Menstrual state and exercise as determinants of spinal bone density in female athletes. *Br Med J* (1990), **301**: 516–8.

25. Spector TD. Use of oestrogen replacement therapy in high risk groups in the United Kingdom. *Br Med J* (1989), **299**: 1433–5.

26. Compston JE, Yamaguchi K, Croucher PI et al. The effect of gonadotrophin-releasing hormone agonists on iliac crest cancellous bone structure in women with endometriosis. *Bone* (1994), **16**: 261–7.

27. Devogelaer JP, Crabbe J, Nagent de Deuxchaines C. Bone mineral density in Addison's disease: evidence for an effect of adrenal androgens on bone mass. *Br Med J* (1987), **294**: 798–800.

28. Melton LJ, Riggs BL. Epidemiology of age-related fractures. In: Alvioli LV ed. *The osteoporotic syndrome*. Grune and Stratton: New York (1983), pp. 45–72.

29. Smith R, Athanasou NA, Ostlere SJ et al. Pregnancy-associated osteoporosis. *Q J Med* (1995), **88**: 865–78.

30. Dunne F, Walters B, Marshall T et al. Pregnancy-associated osteoporosis. *Clin Endocrinol* (1993), **39**: 487–90.

31. Montane de la Roque PH, Cornu JL, Boyer M et al. Spontaneous femoral neck fracture in pregnancy-associated transient regional osteoporosis of the hip. Magnetic resonance imaging findings. *Rev Rhum, Engl edition* (1993), **60**: 452–3.

32. Deodhar AA, Woolf AD. Bone mass measurement and bone metabolism in rheumatoid arthritis: a review. *Br J Rheumatol* (1996), **35**: 309–22.

33. Emery P. The optimal management of early rheumatoid disease: the key to preventing disability. *Br J Rheumatol* (1994), **33**: 765–8.

34. Reid DM, Kennedy NSJ, Smith MA et al. Total body calcium in rheumatoid arthritis: effects of disease activity and corticosteroid treatment. *Br Med J* (1982), **285**: 230–2.

35. Cocksedge S, Freestone S, Martin JF. Unrecognised femoral fractures in patients with paraplegia due to multiple sclerosis. *Br Med J* (1984), **289**: 309.

36. Colver GB, Dawber RPR, Ryan TJ et al. Osteoporosis and mastocytosis with late appearance of urticaria pigmentosa. *J R Soc Med* (1985), **78**: 866–7.

37. Adami S, Fossaluzza V, Gatti D et al. Bisphosphonate therapy of reflex sympathetic dystrophy syndrome. *Ann Rheum Dis* (1997) **56**: 201–4.

38. Markham A, Bryson HM. Deflazacort. A review of its pharmacological properties and therapeutic efficacy. *Drugs* (1995), **50**: 317–33.

39. Lukert BP, Johnson BE, Robinson RG. Estrogen and progesterone replacement therapy reduces glucocorticoid induced bone loss. *J Bone Miner Res* (1992), **7**: 1063–9.

40. Mulder H, Stivis A. Intermittent cyclical etidronate in the prevention of steroid-induced osteoporosis. *Br J Rheumatol* (1994), **33**: 348–50.

41. de Swiet M. Selected side effects: 6. Heparin and osteoporosis. *Prescribers Journal* (1992), **32**: 74–7.

42. Philip WLU, Martin JC, Richardson JM et al. Decreased axial and peripheral bone density in patients taking long-term warfarin. *Q J Med* (1995), **88**: 3635–40.

43. Whitehouse RW, Adams JE, Bancroft K et al. The effects of nafarellin and danazol on vertebral

trabecular bone mass in patients with
endometriosis. *Clin Endocrinol* (1990), **33**: 365–73.

44. Cundy T, Cornish J, Evans MC et al. Recovery of
bone density in women who stop using
medroxyprogesterone acetate. *Br Med J* (1994),
308: 247–8.

45. Lalor BC, France MW, Powell D et al. Bone and
mineral metabolism and chronic alcohol abuse. *Q
J Med* (1986), **59**: 497–512.

46. Holbrook TL, Barrett-Connor E. A prospective
study of alcohol consumption and bone mineral
density. *Br Med J* (1993), **306**: 1506–9.

47. Krall EA, Dawson-Hughes B. Smoking and bone
loss among postmenopausal women. *J Bone Miner
Res* (1991), **6**: 331–7.

48. May H, Murphy S, Khaw K-T. Cigarette smoking
and bone mineral density in older men. *Q J Med*
(1994), **87**: 65.

49. McParland BE, Goulding A, Campbell AJ. Dietary
salt affects biochemical markers of resorption and
formation of bone in elderly women. *Br Med J*
(1989), **299**: 834–5.

50. Iqbal TH, Wood GM, Lewis KO et al. Prevalence of
primary lactase deficiency in adult residents of
West Birmingham. *Br Med J* (1993), **306**: 1303–4.

51. Wheadon M, Goulding A, Barbezat GO et al.
Lactose malabsorption and calcium intake as risk
factors in elderly New Zealand women. *N Z Med
J* (1991), **104**: 417–19.

52. von Wowern N, Klausen B, Olgaard KJ. Steroid-
induced mandibular bone loss in relation to
marginal periodontal changes. *Clin Periodontol*
(1992), **19**: 182–6.

53. Stamp T. Grey hairs, false teeth and bad bones
[Editorial]. *Lancet* (1995), **345**: 876.

54. Galagher SJ, Deighan C, Wallace AM et al.
Association of severe haemophilia A with
osteoporosis: a densitometric and biochemical
study. *Q J Med* (1984), **310**: 1694–6.

55. Paterson CR, McAllion S, Stellman JL.
Osteogenesis imperfecta after the menopause. *N
Engl J Med* (1994), **87**: 181–6.

56. Browner WS, Malinow MR. Homocyst(e)inaemia
and bone density in elderly women. *Lancet* (1991),
338: 1470.

57. Mole PA, Paterson CR. Complete androgen
insensitivity and osteoporosis. (Communication to
the Bone and Tooth Society, Southampton, March
20th 1994.)

58. Levy HL, Driscoll SJ, Pozensky RS. Ovarian
failure in galactosaemia. *N Engl J Med* (1984), **308**:
50–3.

5 Differential diagnosis of bone pain and fracture

INTRODUCTION

The main clinical feature of osteoporosis is susceptibility to fracture, either spontaneously or with minimal trauma, with resultant pain. The main radiological feature is loss of bone mass, osteopenia, perceived as increased bone transradiancy on X-ray, and low scores for bone mineral content on bone density scanning. Osteomalacia and Paget's disease may mimic osteoporosis in the elderly, and osteogenesis imperfecta and fibrous dysplasia of bone may mimic idiopathic and juvenile forms of osteoporosis in younger adults and children. Osteomyelitis of the spine, potentially fatal, may present with a spinal crush fracture. It is important to differentiate these conditions from osteoporosis.

OSTEOMALACIA

Osteomalacia is a delay in, or failure of, mineralization of the bone matrix caused by a lack of vitamin D or disturbance of its metabolism (see Figure 1.14). In the growing skeleton the epiphyses are affected, causing rickets. In adults, the disturbance of bone remodelling is termed osteomalacia. The histological signature of osteomalacia in the bone biopsy is the presence of widened osteoid seams but a presumptive diagnosis can be achieved by other means. Subtypes of osteomalacia and rickets require further investigation to establish their different aetiologies.[1]

Epidemiology

Vitamin D deficiency as a cause of osteomalacia typically occurs in elderly people and in Asians living in northern latitudes. Rickets is occasionally seen in premature infants and may reflect maternal vitamin D depletion or inadequate supplementation of artificial feeds. Routine fortification of infant feeds with vitamin D is dangerous, however.

Causes

Osteomalacia is usually alimentary or renal in origin (see Table 5.1). 1,25-Dihydroxy-vitamin D_3 (calcitriol) is the most potent vitamin D metabolite. The role of 24,25-dihydroxy-vitamin D_3 in mineralization is not yet clearly established (see page 21).[2]

- Parathyroid hormone is raised in vitamin D deficiency and malabsorption, and very high in renal failure but normal or low in hypophosphataemic osteomalacia.

- Osteocalcin levels are normal or slightly raised.

The blood biochemistry is abnormal in most osteomalacic patients. Low serum 25-hydroxy-vitamin D or elevated parathyroid hormone levels may point to dietary deficiency of vitamin D. The diagnosis can only be made with certainty by bone biopsy, however. Urinalysis is an important screen for many of the causes of osteomalacia other than simple vitamin D deficiency.

Table 5.2   Histological features of osteomalacia

		Osteomalacia	Normal
1	Osteoid surfaces with calcification fronts	↓	>60%
2	Osteoid seam thickness	↑	4–13 μm
3	Surfaces covered with osteoid	↑	<24%
4	Bone volume occupied by osteoid	↑	<2%
5	Mineralization rate	↓	0.4–0.7 μm/day
6	Mineralization lag time	↑	<20 days

Histology

Transiliac biopsy following tetracycline labelling, examined by fluorescence microscopy, reveals an abundance of calcification fronts that are not being mineralized. Undecalcified sections cut with a heavy sledge microtome and stained by Von Kossa's method show widened osteoid seams. As a rough guide, osteoid seams wider than a red cell in the same field are abnormal (see Table 5.2 and Figure 5.1).

Radiology

In childhood rickets the growth plates of the long bones show widening and the calcification border becomes ragged and cupped. Bony deformities will also be evident (see Figure 5.2). In adults the characteristic feature is the pseudofracture or Looser's zone (see Figure 5.3). This is a ribbon-like area of rarefaction across the bone, perpendicular to the cortex and initially only extending partially across the width of the bone from the convex side. Such pseudofractures are often bilateral and symmetrical, can occur in almost any bone but are seen most often in those bearing major mechanical stresses. The neck of femur, the pelvis, the pubic ramus, the ribs, the outer borders of the scapulae and the metatarsals are common sites. Generalized osteopenia is usually also present in the elderly and in those with bowel or hepatic disease.

Secondary hyperparathyroidism results in generalized loss of cortical bone. In renal failure this can be severe enough to produce subperiosteal reabsorption of bone in the phalanges, in the pubic symphysis or in the outer ends of the clavicles. Rarely, bone 'cysts' are seen.

The spine may show biconcavity of the vertebral bodies (cod fish vertebrae) (see Figure 5.4). This is different from that seen in osteoporosis as it is regular from bone to bone with normal or increased apparent bone density.

Bone scintiscanning has been shown to predict osteomalacia in an elderly population.[3] There is a generally increased skeletal uptake with 'hot spots' in the ribs or near joints.

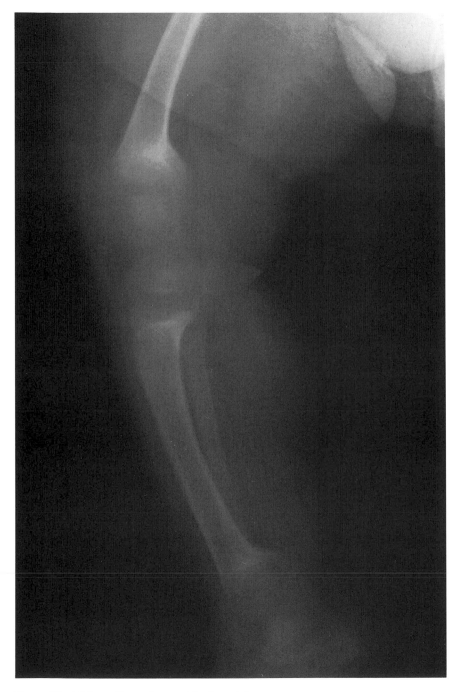

Figure 5.2   Rickets. X-ray shows widening of the
growth plates and curvature of the long bones.

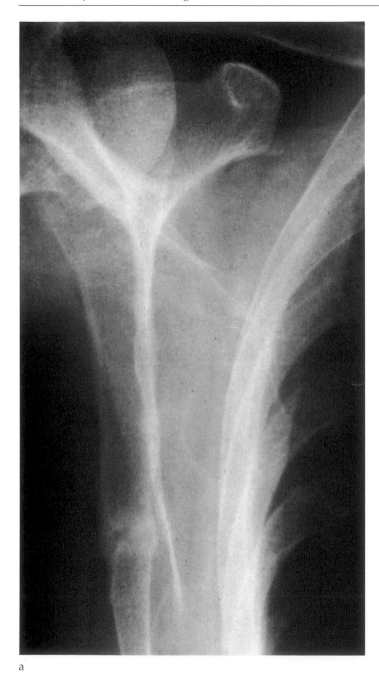

a

Figure 5.3   Pseudofractures or Looser's zones of (a) the lateral border of the scapula and (b) the medial border of the upper femora.

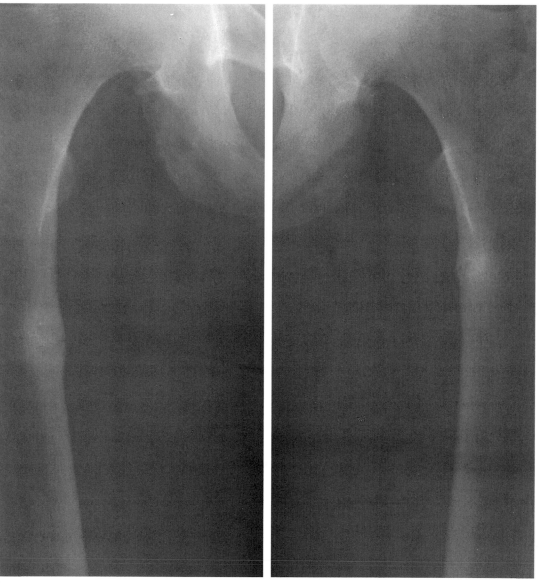

b

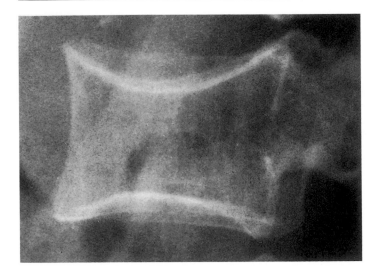

Figure 5.4 Increased biconcavity of the vertebral bodies (cod fish vertebra) is seen in osteomalacia. It is also seen in other causes of bone weakening such as osteoporosis and hyperparathyroidism when the nucleus pulposus is normal, but in osteomalacia adjacent vertebrae are usually affected similarly and the bone density may appear normal. A distinction is not always possible.

Diagnosis

Osteomalacia needs to be distinguished from:

- other osteopenic conditions;
- other causes of proximal weakness such as polymyalgia rheumatica, thyrotoxic myopathy, hypothyroidism, muscular dystrophy, carcinomatous neuromyopathy, dermatomyositis and polymyositis;
- other causes of bone pain such as Paget's disease, multiple myeloma, leukaemia and prostatic or breast carcinomatosis;
- other causes of pain and stiffness on movement, especially osteoarthritis of the hips and polymyalgia rheumatica.

Plasma calcium, phosphate and alkaline phosphatase levels should identify patients who have osteomalacia, but failing this bone biopsy will show the characteristic histological features. In vitamin D deficiency, plasma vitamin D levels and parathyroid hormone levels, if available, are helpful.

Treatment

There is a rapid response to vitamin D. Muscle weakness is the first symptom to respond but bone pain may temporarily increase. Increasing calcium and phosphate absorption is the first biochemical responses. Paradoxically, the plasma alkaline phosphatase level and urinary hydroxyproline output may temporarily rise, falling slowly to normal. As the plasma 25-hydroxy-vitamin D and calcium levels normalize, PTH falls. Healing of bone takes several months and dietary supplements of calcium and phosphate are essential.

The effective dose and the choice of which derivative of vitamin D to use depend on the cause of the osteomalacia. The dose will have to be adjusted depending on serum levels of calcium, phosphatase, alkaline phosphatase and vitamin D.

- Vitamin D deficiency responds to UV light or 1500–5000 IU/day orally or 10 000–50 000 IU/month intramuscularly of ergocalciferol (calciferol, vitamin D_2) with adequate calcium and phosphate intake. Alternatively, 1,25-dihydroxy-vitamin D_3 (calcitriol, initially 250 ng daily or alternate days increasing to 0.5–1 µg daily) or 1-α-hydroxycholecalciferol (alfacalcidol, initially 1 µg daily with a maintenance of 0.25–1 µg daily) can be used. Vitamin D_2 is inexpensive and has a long half-life.

- The initial treatment of osteomalacia in chronic renal failure requires up to 3 µg of calcitriol or 1 µg of alfacalcidol daily, with monitoring of plasma calcium. For a maintenance or prophylactic treatment only about 0.5 µg daily is required.
- Renal tubular disorders are treated by correcting the acidosis, and giving an adequate phosphate intake of 1–2 g per day and small doses of calcitriol or alfacalcidol.
- Hypophosphataemic osteomalacia is treated with 1–5 µg of calcitriol or alfacalcidol and 1–4 g/day phosphate supplements, with careful monitoring for hypercalcaemia.

MYELOMA AND METASTATIC CANCER

Causes

The commonest primary malignant tumour of bone is multiple myeloma. The skeleton is also the commonest nonlymphatic site of metastatic deposits from carcinomata and sarcomata. The bones affected, in order of frequency, are the vertebrae, proximal femur, pelvis, ribs, sternum and proximal humerus. Cancers which commonly metastasize to bone include those of the prostate, breast, lung, thyroid, kidney and bladder.

Osteolytic metastases predispose to fracture and arise from thyroid, kidney, lower bowel and most breast carcinomata. Osteosclerotic metastases characteristically derive from carcinoma of the prostate. Carcinoid, Hodgkin's disease and breast carcinomata are rarer causes.

Cancer cells produce factors that increase osteoclastic activity, producing osteolysis and hypercalcaemia. Other cancers and the multiple endocrine neoplasia syndrome may give rise to osteopenia by producing prostaglandins or PTH-like factors or hypercortisolaemia.[4]

Signs and symptoms

Some bony lesions are clinically silent and detected only by the discovery of hypercalcaemia, or by skeletal survey or by scintiscans. Other lesions give rise to pain, swelling, deformity, leucoerythroblastic anaemia from marrow invasion, spinal cord or nerve root compression, or to pathological fractures. Hypercalcaemia can cause loss of appetite, polyuria, nocturia and polydipsia, and depression. Patients with serious hypercalcaemia may even go into coma or develop secondary renal shut-down.

Biochemistry

Hypercalcaemia

Cancer and hyperparathyroidism are the commonest causes of hypercalcaemia,[5] the former being more common in hospital in-patient surveys and the latter in population surveys. The causes of hypercalcaemia are shown in Table 5.3. The diagnosis of underlying malignant disease is shown in Table 5.4. Hypercalcaemia is only rarely associated with tumours not invading bone.

Metastatic disease is usually apparent before presentation with hypercalcaemia. The serum

Table 5.3 Causes of hypercalcaemia

- Malignancy
  Lytic bone metastases
  Ectopic production of 1,25-dihydroxy-vitamin D_3 (lymphomas)
  PTH-related protein (carcinoma of lung, oesophagus, head and neck, kidney, ovary and bladder)
  Other factor(s) produced locally or ectopically
- Hyperparathyroidism
  Primary
  Associated with chronic renal failure
- Vitamin D intoxication
- Sarcoidosis
- Thyrotoxicosis
- Hypoalbuminaemia
- Immobilization
- Milk–alkali syndrome
- Infantile hypercalcaemia, idiopathic or related to vitamin D fortification of infant feeds
- Acute renal failure (polyuric recovery phase)
- Familial hypocalciuric hypercalcaemia
- Addison's disease
- Thiazide diuretics, especially in dehydrated patients
- Rare
  Tuberculosis
  Phaeochromocytoma
  Vasoactive intestinal polypeptide-secreting tumour (vipoma)
  Acromegaly
  Lithium treatment
  Total parental nutrition
  Coccidioidomycosis
  Berylliosis
  Manganese intoxication
  Hypereosinophilic syndrome
  Hypothyroidism
  Vitamin A poisoning
  Benign breast hyperplasia

Table 5.4 Malignant disease as a cause of hypercalcaemia

	No. of patients	% of cases
Malignant disease	72	100
of which Lung	25	35
Breast	18	25
Haematologic (Myeloma 5, Lymphoma 4)	10	14
Head and Neck	4	6
Renal	2	3
Prostate	2	3
Unknown primary	5	7
Others (GI tract, 4)	8	9

Adapted from Mundy GR, and Martin TJ, 1982[5]

Radiology

The patient may have the typical punched-out lesions of myeloma (see Figure 5.5 and case history below), which need differentiating from hyperparathyroidism. Alternatively, there may be a marked sclerotic response (see Figure 5.6), which needs to be differentiated from Paget's disease. The most effective method for identifying skeletal metastases is radioisotope scanning (see Figure 5.7), although infection, trauma and benign tumours may appear as areas of increased isotope uptake. False negative scans occur in myeloma.

calcium is usually normal or low with osteosclerotic metastases. The serum alkaline phosphatase is characteristically elevated with osteosclerotic lesions but may be normal with some osteolytic lesions, particularly with myeloma.

> Mrs C W developed polymyalgia rheumatica at the age of 63 years and was maintained on low-dose prednisolone (2–4 mg per day). At 74 years of age increased stoop and back pain were noted. Investigations revealed an elevated erythrocyte sedimentation rate, and protein electrophoresis showed monoclonal gammopathy. Bence-Jones protein was detected in the urine. X-rays showed spinal crush fractures.

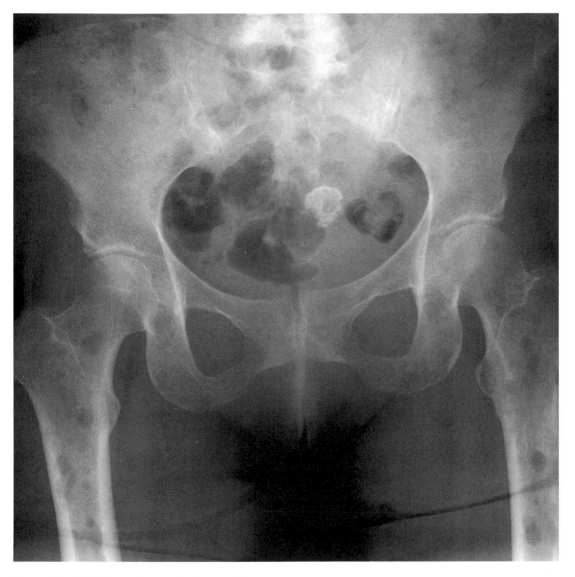

Figure 5.5 Multiple myeloma with characteristic 'punched out' lytic lesions most apparent in the upper femora.

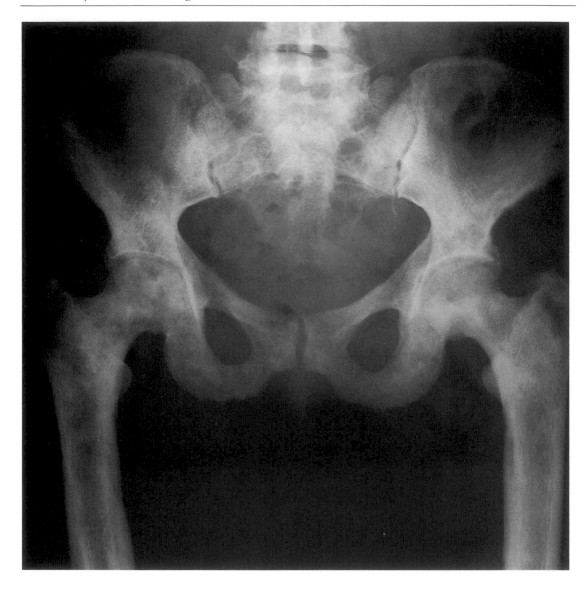

Figure 5.6 Sclerotic and lytic metastases of
carcinoma of the breast, giving a similar appearance
to Paget's disease.

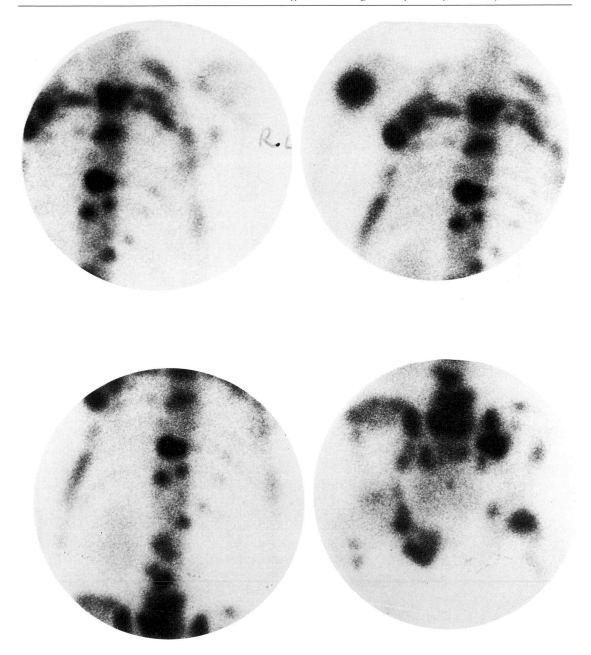

Figure 5.7   Metastases of a carcinoma of prostate demonstrated by increased tracer uptake.

Other investigations

Myeloma is characterized by greatly increased sedimentation rate and plasma viscosity, and raised serum globulin, and also by the presence of a monoclonal gammopathy with the detection of lambda or kappa light chains in the urine. A primary cancer is usually evident but, if the patient presents with asymptomatic hypercalcaemia, the differential diagnosis is most commonly between cancer, hyperparathyroidism, vitamin D intoxication, and less commonly sarcoidosis (Table 5.3). The level of serum PTH (best measured by immunoradiometric assay (IRMA)) is the best means of differentiating hyperparathyroidism, although a failure to suppress calcium levels with corticosteroids should help (see page 142). In some cancer patients hypercalcaemia may persist despite glucocorticoid therapy. Serum parathyroid hormone related protein (PTHRP), which is not detected by IRMA, may be responsible for tumoral hypercalcaemia, indicated by abnormally low levels of IRMA or by specific tests for PTHRP.

Treatment

Control of the malignancy by either chemotherapy or radiotherapy usually results in a fall in the serum calcium and symptomatic improvement. Sometimes hypercalcaemia will need direct management.

A serum calcium level above 12 mg/dl (3 mmol/litre) warrants urgent intervention, irrespective of signs, symptoms or the eventual diagnosis.

- The priority is to give intravenous normal saline taking care not to produce hypokalaemia or fluid overload. This will rehydrate and enhance urinary calcium excretion. A loop diuretic may sometimes be used to inhibit sodium and calcium resorption, but only when extracellular fluid volume has been replenished.

- A slow intravenous infusion of a bisphosphonate should be given. Suitable formulations include disodium etidronate (50 mg/ml, 7.5 mg/kg body weight daily over two to four hours for three days, repeat at intervals of seven days if necessary), disodium pamidronate (3 mg/ml, 15–60 mg by slow infusion) or sodium clodronate (30 mg/ml, 300 mg daily for up to 10 days).

- Systemic glucocorticoids are effective but are too slow for emergency treatment. Prednisolone is given, commencing with 40–60 mg daily and reducing according to response. Calcitonin alone is not very effective but may be potent in combination with glucocorticoids especially when treating haematological malignancies.

- Dialysis against a low-calcium dialysate is usually reserved for severe hypercalcaemia.

- Plicamycin, previously called mithramycin, inhibits bone resorption and effectively lowers elevated calcium levels in most patients. It is given intravenously in a dose of 15–25 μg/kg over four to six hours. It has considerable toxicity, which limits its usefulness. It remains a reasonable choice to correct hypercalcaemia rapidly.

PAGET'S DISEASE

Paget's disease is characterized by excessive bone resorption coupled with increased but disorganized bone formation. Interest in this condition has increased since the introduction of effective treatments and evidence that it might be caused by a slow virus infection.[6]

Epidemiology

The prevalence varies geographically. It is common in the UK, Australia, New Zealand,

Central Europe and in the USA, but is rare in Scandinavia, Africa and the Middle and Far East. Judged radiologically, it affects about 4% of the population over 40 years old in the UK, increasing to 10% in very elderly people. Clinically, however, only one in twenty of these will have symptoms.

Cause

Is Paget's disease of viral origin? Tubulofilamentous paracrystalline particles have been identified within the nuclei and the cytoplasm of osteoclasts from affected bone. These inclusions are not found in the osteoclasts of normal bone from patients with Paget's disease, nor in the osteoclasts of patients with primary or secondary hyperparathyroidism. They have the characteristics of nucleocapsids of the *Paramyxovirus* family, in particular of respiratory syncytial virus, and may represent a slow virus infection such as the measles-like *Paramyxovirus* which is thought to cause sclerosing panencephalitis. Antigens of both respiratory syncytial virus and measles virus have been found in osteoclasts and mononuclear cells cultured from Pagetic bone. So far, neither isolation of this putative virus nor its transmission to animals has been reported. The question also remains whether this particle may be a passenger rather than a cause of the disease. However, the infective nature of Paget's disease is supported by natural autograft experiments. When normal bone is used to graft vertebral bone affected by Paget's disease, for example to repair spinal defects caused by operations to relieve spinal stenosis, the graft is invaded by the Paget's process. The graft does not grow into and normalize the Paget's bone.

There is an increased number of osteoclasts that are larger than normal and have more nuclei. Hence, the initial phase of Paget's disease is net bone resorption and affected bones appear osteoporotic. This is followed by an active osteoblastic and sclerotic phase with the formation of excess woven bone. Then there is a quiescent phase. In multifocal disease sufferers may demonstrate all phases occurring at once in different bones. Affected bones become extremely vascular and an increase in intramedullary pressure is thought to be one cause of pain in Paget's disease. This vascularity may also lead to increased blood loss at surgery.

Signs and symptoms

Pain

This is the commonest presenting complaint and may affect any bone. There are several causes. When due to Pagetic changes, it is characterized by a deep nagging pain which is worse at night, unrelated to activity and variable in severity. Involvement of the bones of the face and jaw (leontiasis ossea) is particularly liable to cause pain. Partial fractures, which only affect the convex aspects of the long bones, may also be painful. Complete fractures of the long bones with little or no trauma also occur during the lytic phase and there is often nonunion. Radicular pain due to spinal root compression occurs, while pain may also arise from distorted joints and secondary osteoarthritis, or there may be coincidental osteoarthritic changes. Painful osteoarthritis may be distinguished from pain arising directly from Pagetic-diseased bone by the response to calcitonin or bisphosphonates.

Deformity

Affected bones become thicker. This is most obvious in the limbs and skull, and leads to nerve entrapment, deafness and osteoarthritic changes in the joints. Spinal involvement may lead to collapse fractures of vertebral bodies, loss of height, marked transverse abdominal creases and ribs that rest on the pelvic rim as in osteoporosis. Spinal collapse in Paget's disease may result in paraplegia, which is exceedingly rare in osteoporosis.

Neurological

Nerves may be involved in Paget's disease of the skull and vertebral column. Early localized involvement of the skull is seen as a lucent zone, osteoporosis circumscripta. Later, the skull X-ray has a 'cotton wool' appearance due to osteolytic and reparative disease. Headaches are a common complaint at this stage. Basilar invagination may produce vertebrobasilar insufficiency, cerebellar signs, brain stem compression or internal hydrocephalus. Deafness is the commonest complication of skull involvement in Paget's disease, occurring in up to 50% of sufferers. When the petrous temporal bones are involved the vestibular apparatus or the auditory nerve itself can suffer compression. In others, the ossicles of the inner ear are involved.

Cardiovascular system

In widespread 'active' Paget's disease, the cardiac output is increased but heart failure is rare. The increased blood flow is the first morbid physiological manifestation of Paget's disease to respond to treatment and in surface bones is detectable by reduced heat flux on thermography. Increased blood flow to the skull may cause a 'steal' syndrome, with the patient suffering drop attacks similar to those in vertebrobasilar insufficiency.

Paget's sarcoma

This occurs in less than 1% of all patients, but the frequency rises to 20% in those who have suffered from symptomatic Paget's disease for 20 years or more. The pelvis, femur and then the humerus are the commonest sites of malignant transformation. Those at high risk include patients with polyostotic disease and those with disease of the humerus (which is not the commonest site of Paget's disease). Two-thirds of the neoplasms are osteosarcomata and the others are either fibrosarcomata or occasionally chondrosarcomata. They present with worsening of bone pain, pathological fractures or a sudden increase of plasma alkaline phosphatase which does not respond to treatment. The prognosis is poor.

Biochemistry

Biochemical changes reflect the increase in bone resorption and formation. Although these rates may be increased up to fortyfold, there is usually little disturbance in serum calcium and phosphate levels and urinary calcium output. If something else upsets the linkage between formation and resorption, such as fracture or immobilization, patients show a negative calcium balance with an increase in serum calcium and urine calcium output.

The alkaline phosphatase level, of osteoblastic origin, increases. Sometimes this is within the normal range, but will fall with treatment, suggesting that it is elevated for that individual. Alkaline phosphatase has a short half-life and therefore rapidly reflects changes in osteoblastic activity. The increased level in Paget's disease corresponds to the extent and activity of the disease and correlates with radiological and bone scanning assessment of skeletal involvement. It also correlates closely with the urinary hydroxyproline output, deoxypyridinoline cross-links and N-telopeptides, which are measures of bone collagen resorption, thus showing the close coupling between bone formation and resorption. The greatly increased bone mineral turnover in 'active' Paget's disease may be reflected in non-Paget's bone as widened osteoid seams (i.e., in mild to moderate osteomalacia).

Urinary hydroxyproline excretion is increased in active disease. The most abundant source of this is collagen and 90% of that found in the urine is derived from collagen degradation. It correlates with plasma alkaline phosphatase and radiological assessment of bony involvement. Dietary collagen contributes to this, but this effect is avoided by assaying an early morning fasting sample and expressing the results in terms of the hydroxyproline:creatinine ratio. This and newer biochemical markers of bone resorption, urinary collagen cross-links, may serve as rapid measures and predictors of response to treatment (see page 75).

Radiology

Changes may be either osteolytic or osteosclerotic (see Figures 5.8 and 5.9). Osteolytic lesions usually begin at one end of long bones and progress down the shaft, advancing as fast as 1 cm per year. Osteosclerotic changes result in remodelling of the bone, with expansion and disorganization of the architecture and loss of the normal trabecular pattern. The overall size of bones increases. Coexisting zones of rarefaction and sclerosis may be seen.

Scintiscanning may show areas of increased skeletal vascularity and turnover where there are only minimal radiological changes.

Diagnosis

This is made by a combination of radiology, scanning and biochemistry. X-rays of the lumbosacral spine, pelvis and upper femurs will identify most cases.

Treatment

Indications

- Pain
- Major osteolytic lesions in weight-bearing bones, at risk of fracture
- Neurological complications
- Prior to and following orthopaedic surgery
- Fracture
- Hypercalcaemia
- Increased cardiac output.

Nonspecific therapy

Orthopaedic appliances, shoe modifications and hearing aids may be helpful. Surgery may be required for fractures, or arthroplasties for secondary osteoarthritis. Mild to moderate non-opiate analgesics or nonsteroidal anti-inflammatory drugs are often effective for pain. Occasionally, especially in Paget's disease of the facial bones (leontiasis ossea) or in Paget's sarcoma, strong analgesics such as methadone or morphine will be required.

Specific therapy

Two groups of drugs are now available: calcitonins and bisphosphonates.

Calcitonins (see also Chapter 9, page 217)

Human calcitonin is a 32-amino acid polypeptide hormone that inhibits bone resorption by reducing osteoclastic activity. Synthetic forms of salmon calcitonin (salcatonin) and synthetic analogues of eel (elcatonin) and genetically engineered human calcitonin are available. Bone pain and temperature measured thermographically are rapidly reduced and the serum alkaline phosphatase and urinary hydroxyproline output fall to 50% of pretreatment levels but often remain abnormal, increasing when treatment ceases.

A dose of 50–100 IU of calcitonin should be given subcutaneously initially daily and after

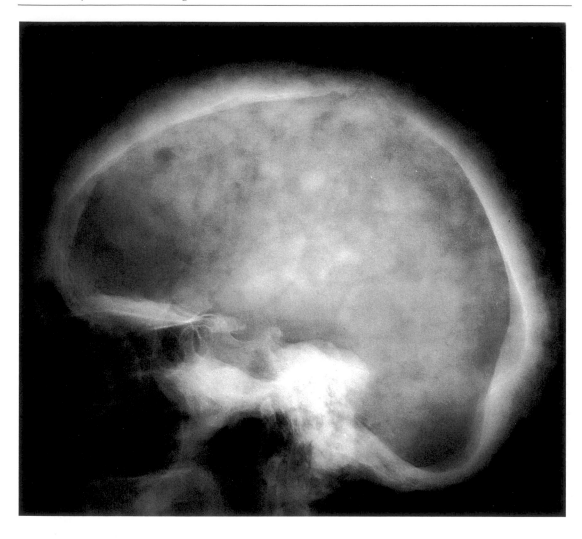

a

Figure 5.8   Paget's disease of the (a,b) skull, (c)
pelvis and proximal femur and (d) of a single
vertebra which has collapsed.

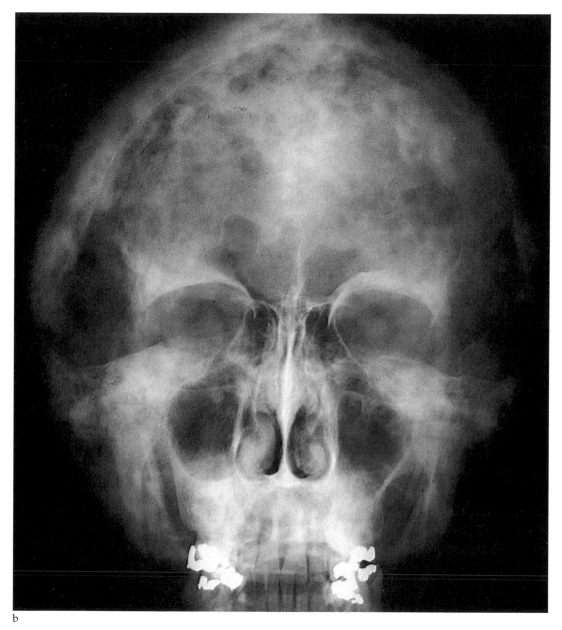

b

b

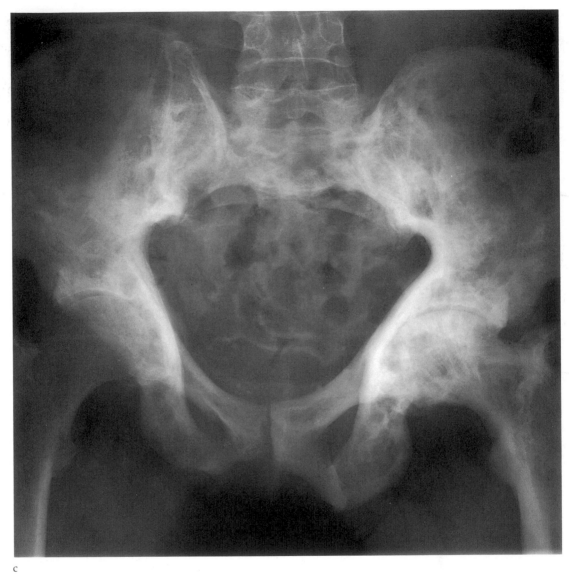

c

c

Figure 5.8 *continued*

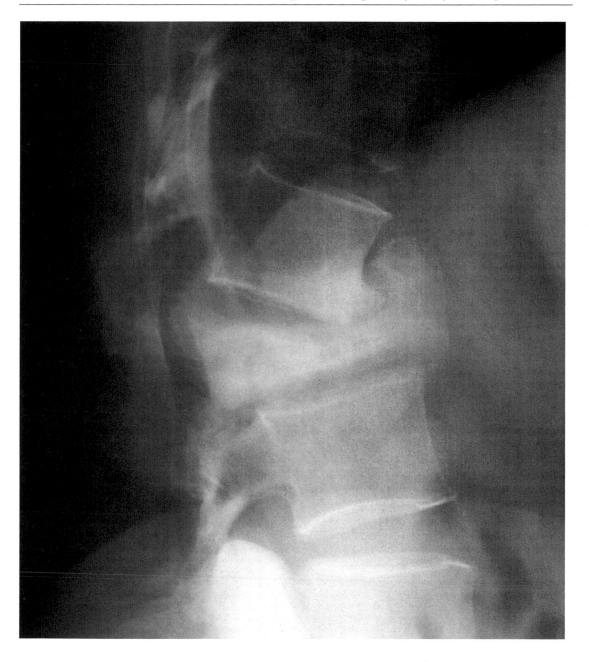

d

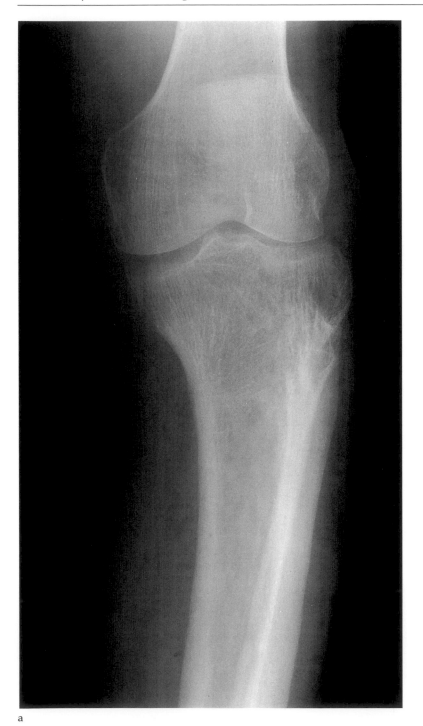

a

Figure 5.9 (a) Paget's disease of the tibia with widening and bowing. (b) The increased vascularity is demonstrated by increased temperature as measured by infrared thermography.

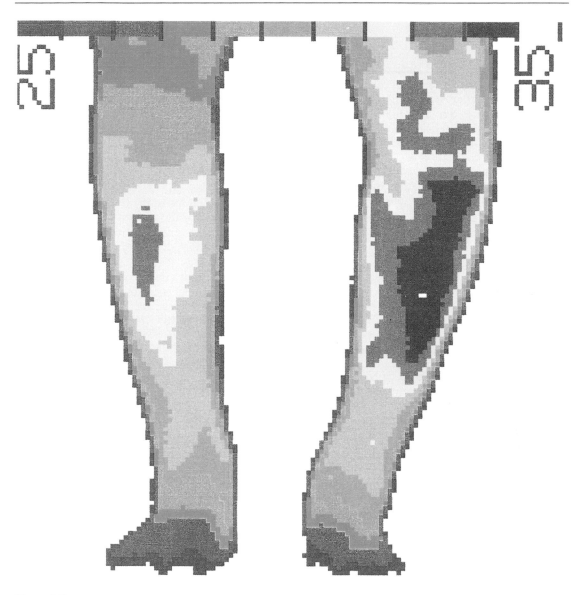

Figure 5.9b

three months, when there is usually a biochemical response, it can be given two to three times a week for six to twelve months. Patients can be re-treated if necessary. There is a 30% relapse rate within one year and 25% of patients develop resistance. Although the latter is not always due to antibody formation, it is worthwhile trying calcitonin from a different species. X-ray healing has been seen. The main adverse effect is nausea; less often there is facial flushing, tingling of the extremities, itching, fever and a metallic taste in the mouth. These all settle after a few weeks of continuous treatment. Because of its expense, calcitonin has generally been superseded by the bisphosphonates.

Bisphosphonates (see also Chapter 9, page 218)

These are analogues of pyrophosphate in which the labile P–O–P bond has been changed to a stable P–C–P bond. Most experience has been gained with disodium etidronate, the first to be licensed for the treatment of Paget's disease, but all bisphosphonates have similar effects. They inhibit both the growth and dissolution of hydroxyapatite crystals in vitro and retard bone resorption and bone formation in animals. They are taken up by bone and are poorly released. Intestinal absorption is poor, varying between 1% and 5%, and this is decreased by calcium and magnesium ions in the gastric contents. They should therefore be taken on an empty stomach.

A dose of 5 mg/kg per day (400 mg per day in most patients) of disodium etidronate is effective for the symptomatic, biochemical and histological suppression of Paget's disease. High doses, however, are associated with increased risk of fracture due to defective mineralization. Etidronate should be given for six months and the improvement may persist for years. Treatment may be repeated if required, and some patients follow six months

on, six months off cycles with long-term benefit. Combination therapy with calcitonin has been used and might give a better response. Side-effects include diarrhoea, hyperphosphataemia and excessive osteoid. Some patients respond poorly and, on X-ray, bones may appear osteoporotic with an unchecked advance of the 'Paget's front' into the normal bone. Close and frequent radiological and biochemical supervision therefore is advisable.

Newer bisphosphonates are more potent and have little effect on mineralization at doses used to inhibit bone resorption. Patients should have vitamin D and calcium supplements to avoid hypocalcaemia in the early phase of treatment with a potent bisphosphonate.

Pamidronate is a potent bisphosphonate (see Chapter 9) that is given by intravenous infusion. Various regimes are used to treat Paget's disease: one being 30 mg infusions given weekly for six weeks. Infusions should be given slowly.

Alendronate is a potent orally administered aminobisphosphonate and 40 mg daily for six months is recommended. It should be taken on rising in the morning before any food, drink or other tablets with at least 8 oz tap water. No food or drink other than tap water should be taken for at least 30 minutes otherwise absorption will be minimal and during this time the patient should stand or sit upright as recumbency after swallowing the drug has been associated with oesophagitis.

Tiludronate is an orally administered bisphosphonate licenced for the treatment of Paget's disease. It is well tolerated and given as 400 mg daily for 12 weeks. It should be taken at a minimum of 2 hours before and after food, with water. Risedronate and ibandronate are under development. They are 3000–5000 times more potent than etidronate and the therapeutic margin is favourable. Ibandronate promises to be able to be given by intravenous injection at up to 3-monthly intervals. It may be effective as medicated adhesive patches. Studies in Paget's disease are awaited.

There is a long-lasting response to these newer bisphosphonates in most patients.

HYPERPARATHYROIDISM

Primary hyperparathyroidism was originally recognized in association with osteitis fibrosa cystica but other manifestations of the disease are more common.

Epidemiology

Less severe forms of the disease are now recognized. Routine biochemical screening for raised PTH or calcium levels identifies up to 50% of patients; up to 30% of all patients are asymptomatic. The prevalence of clinical hyperparathyroidism is between one and three per 1000, with an annual incidence of about 25 per 100 000 population. Primary hyperparathyroidism is approximately twice as common in women than in men.

Pathophysiology

Primary hyperparathyroidism reflects excess secretion of PTH and its fragments. By stimulating renal 1-α-hydroxylase, the production of 1,25-dihydroxy-vitamin D_3 from 25-hydroxy-vitamin D is increased, leading to increased intestinal absorption of calcium. Parathyroid hormone also stimulates the renal resorption of calcium from the glomerular filtrate and the resorption of bone. Excessive production of PTH is caused by a single adenoma in 80–90% of the patients, by multiple adenomata in 2% and by hyperplasia in 5% (the latter group often have a family history of hyperparathyroidism). Hyperparathyroidism may be part of a multiple endocrine adenomatosis ('apudoma'). A PTH-secreting carcinoma is seen in 1–2% of patients. In these, bone disease is frequent, there is often a mass in the neck and recurrence can follow surgery. Secondary hyperparathyroidism may follow prolonged hypocalcaemia in renal failure or steatorrhoea.

Bone histology is nearly always abnormal in primary hyperparathyroidism, although clinical bone disease tends mainly to occur in those with the largest parathyroid tumours and most marked hypercalcaemia. There is evidence of increased bone resorption with prominent osteoclasts and Howship's lacunae on the surface of the trabeculae, which become surrounded by fibrous tissue. Often there is also an increase in osteoblastic activity and there may be new bone formation on one side of a trabeculum with increased osteoclastic resorption on the other side. Osteoid excess is common. As severity increases the marrow space becomes filled with fibrous tissue and the normal structure of the cortex and medulla is replaced by a fine meshwork of irregular trabeculae, suggesting rapid bone formation. The bone is more liable to fracture. Cystic spaces form within the loose vascular fibrous tissue and give the radiological feature of osteitis fibrosa cystica and the histological features of 'brown tumours of hyperparathyroidism'.

Signs and symptoms

Many asymptomatic patients are now detected by biochemical screening. The commonest clinical manifestation is renal colic due to calculi, which is two to three times more common than bone pain, although radiological abnormalities are more common than symptoms. Approximately one-quarter of patients have radiological skeletal changes.

The patient may present with difficulty in walking or climbing stairs, or a waddling gait similar to that seen in osteomalacia. Involvement of joints may also affect mobility, joint disease in hyperparathyroidism taking several forms. Acute crystal synovitis may be caused by urate crystals (gout) or by calcium pyrophosphate crystals (pseudogout), and mixed crystal deposition also occurs. Osteoarthritis is seen, associated with the deposition of calcium pyrophosphate crystals in articular cartilage (chondrocalcinosis). A subacute synovitis resembling rheumatoid arthritis, also with calcium pyrophosphate crystal deposition, is rare. Subchondral bone erosions can lead to collapse and fragmentation of articular bone and distortion of the joint. Hyperparathyroidism is associated with a low bone mass.

Patients may also present with nonspecific symptoms of hypercalcaemia. The commonest is lethargy, while gastrointestinal symptoms, nausea, vomiting, anorexia and weight loss, and constipation, also occur. Hypercalcaemia may cause a nephrogenic diabetes insipidus-like syndrome, with polyuria, nocturia and polydipsia. Psychological changes may occur and some patients are erroneously admitted to mental hospitals. 'Stones, groans and bones' succinctly describes these various presentations.

Conditions associated with primary hyperparathyroidism include peptic ulceration, pancreatitis, pancreatic calcification and hypertension. Renal calculus formation may lead to infection, and pyelonephritis in an elderly woman should always suggest hyperparathyroidism until proved otherwise. Renal tubular dysfunction also leads to urate retention, so that some patients, usually men, present with acute gout.

Biochemistry

- The serum calcium is elevated in all patients. (Blood should be drawn without using a venous tourniquet.) Rarely, this can be intermittently within the normal range. It is important to correct for serum albumin.

- The serum phosphate would be expected to be low considering the effect of PTH, but this is so in less than 50% of patients.

- The serum alkaline phosphatase is slightly elevated in proportion to bone disease and is normal in the majority of cases.

- The daily urinary calcium output is raised.

- Urinary hydroxyproline may be elevated and this is in proportion to the alkaline phosphatase, illustrating the increase in both bone resorption and formation.

- There may also be a mild hyperchloraemic acidosis and a generalized aminoaciduria.

- 1,25-Dihydroxy-vitamin D_3 may be raised due to the stimulation of renal-α-hydroxylase by PTH if renal function is normal.

- Parathyroid hormone is elevated in all patients. Several immunoassays of differing sensitivities are available for measurement. Immunoradiometric assay (IRMA) of PTH detects 80% of sufferers and distinguishes hypercalcaemia in primary hyperparathyroidism from other causes where PTH secretion is suppressed. It is helpful in the localization of an adenoma by selective venous sampling.

- Renal function is impaired in about one-third of patients, more often in those presenting with bone disease than with renal calculus.

Radiology

Diagnostic features are found in about 20% of patients (see Figure 5.10). Subperiosteal erosions are the commonest of these and are best seen on the middle phalanges, especially the radial border of the index finger. Disappearance of the lamina dura, the bone surrounding the roots of teeth, may also be an early feature. Subperiosteal erosions occur in other sites, such as the ends of the clavicles, in the pelvis at the sacroiliac joint or pubic symphysis and the upper tibiae. Cysts may also be found at various sites, including the long bones and the skull. These erosions and cysts heal following parathyroidectomy but the cortex may remain irregular. A few patients present with generalized osteopenia. Bone mass is reduced preferentially at cortical sites with reduction in bone density at the distal third of the forearm with relative preservation of the lumbar spine. Recovery of bone density follows successful treatment.

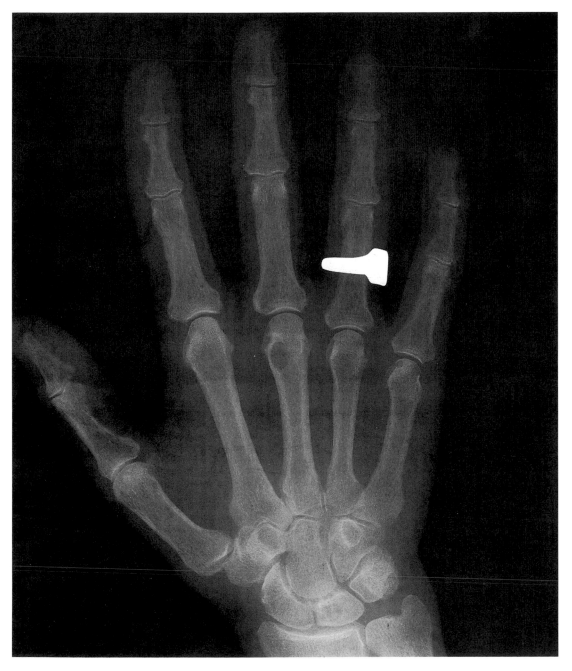

Figure 5.10 Primary hyperparathyroidism.
Subperiosteal erosions can be seen on the radial
border of the second and third middle phalanges and
a bone cyst in the third metacarpal bone.

Diagnosis

Patients may present with renal calculi (30%) or bone pain (15%) but diagnosis is increasingly discovered by biochemical screening when seeking medical care for other reasons. Once hypercalcaemia has been confirmed, other causes need to be excluded, of which malignancy is the most important (Table 5.3). If biochemical features are supported by radiological evidence of hyperparathyroidism then the diagnosis is definite. In other patients assays of immunoreactive PTH are used, as PTH is suppressed in hypercalcaemia of malignancy, and the only hypercalcaemic disorders in which PTH might be elevated are those related to lithium or thiazide diuretic use. In a patient with primary hyperparathyroidism one must also consider the possibility of the multiple endocrine adenoma syndrome (Type I) and look for lesions of the anterior pituitary, parathyroid glands, pancreatic islets and adrenal cortex.

Treatment

Primary hyperparathyroidism is cured by removal of the abnormal parathyroid tissue but the majority of patients are asymptomatic. Surgery is indicated if there are any complications of primary hyperparathyroidism such as overt bone disease, renal calculi or psychiatric manifestations. Surgery is also considered if there is symptomatic hypercalcaemia or the serum calcium is high (> 2.85 mmol/l corrected). Other indications in asymptomatic patients are impaired renal function (creatinine clearance < 30% for age), hypercalcuria (> 400 mg/day), bone mass at distal radius more than 2 standard deviations below age- and sex-matched controls, and in a relatively young patient (under 50 years old) as they have greater long-term risks. About half the patients with primary hyperparathyroidism will meet at least one of these criteria. Surgery to remove these adenomata requires expertise and experience to gain successful results. Preoperative and intraoperative investigations which are used to localize the abnormal parathyroid tissue include ultrasonography, computerized tomography, magnetic resonance imaging, and scintigraphy. Sampling from the branches of the thyroid veins and performing immunoradiometric assay on the serum can also be used. At operation, the adenoma is excised but if all four glands are hyperplastic all but one-third of one gland is removed.

Where surgery is not indicated, then the patient should maintain adequate hydration, avoid thiazide diuretics, and avoid excessive dietary or supplemental calcium. In postmenopausal women hormone replacement therapy will often normalize the serum calcium and restore bone mass.[7] Patients should be reviewed regularly with serum calcium measurement six monthly, and yearly urinary calcium excretion tests and bone density assessment. In most patients mild primary hyperparathyroidism follows a benign course.

OSTEOGENESIS IMPERFECTA

This is a rare and heterogeneous group of congenital disorders, the features of which include fractures due to increased bone fragility, bone pain with or without fracture, skeletal deformities and osteoporosis.[8] Almost all are expressions of congenital and usually autosomal dominant genetic abnormalities of Type I collagen fibres, which in some represent new mutations.[9]

Epidemiology

The prevalence is between one in 20 000 and one in 50 000. A spectrum of severity is seen which represents different biochemical entities

Table 5.5   Classification of osteogenesis imperfecta[10]

Type I: Autosomal dominant

Features are: height normal, deformity unusual; fractures infrequent; bluish sclerae in childhood; hearing loss as young adults in 30%; affected women may have first fractures around the time of the menopause; teeth normal or opalescent.

Type II: Lethal perinatal. Autosomal dominant. (New mutation.)

Features are: intrauterine fractures; soft skull; multiple deformities; if born alive, fatal in first weeks of life.

Type III: Autosomal dominant or recessive

Features are: frequent fractures in childhood leading to deformities, often severe; short stature; blue sclerae in infancy.

Type IV: Autosomal dominant

Features are: mild disease; normal sclerae; dentinogenesis imperfecta; hearing loss common; some skeletal deformity.

Table 5.6   Osteogenesis imperfecta: clinical features

- Osteoporosis
- Fragile bones
- Skeletal deformity
- Blue sclerae
- Deafness
- Abnormal teeth
- Lax ligaments
- Hypermobile joints
- Thin skin
- Cardiac abnormalities

as yet not fully defined. Different families seem to have their own private genetic abnormalities. Clinical classifications (Table 5.5) are unsatisfactory, but all divide a dominantly inherited mild group with prominent extraskeletal features from a rare, heterogeneous, usually autosomal recessive, severe group.

Signs and symptoms

The severe forms are readily apparent, with severe skeletal deformity.

In the milder forms, a painful fracture is the usual presenting manifestation, although pain may occur in the absence of a fracture. Multiple fractures lead to angulations and bowing of the long bones. Vertebral bodies become biconcave and shorten the spine. The pelvis may become deformed with protrusio acetabuli. (Other features are listed in Table 5.6.) Blue sclerae, which are are the only sign of disease in 10% of patients, also occur in hypophosphatasia, Marfan's syndrome and Ehlers–Danlos syndrome. Deafness is the only overt feature in some. Dentinogenesis imperfecta, if present, is seen as small, malaligned, brittle, discoloured teeth. Weakness of collagen in the heart can lead to dilatation of the aortic root, floppy heart valves, ruptured chordae tendineae and cystic medionecrosis of the aorta. Although progressive, osteogenesis imperfecta in those who survive infancy is rarely fatal.

Biochemistry

The serum calcium and phosphate levels are normal, though the serum alkaline phosphatase may be elevated following a fracture. The urinary hydroxyproline output may be increased.

Radiology

There is a wide spectrum ranging from a few fractures of normal bone to multiple fractures,

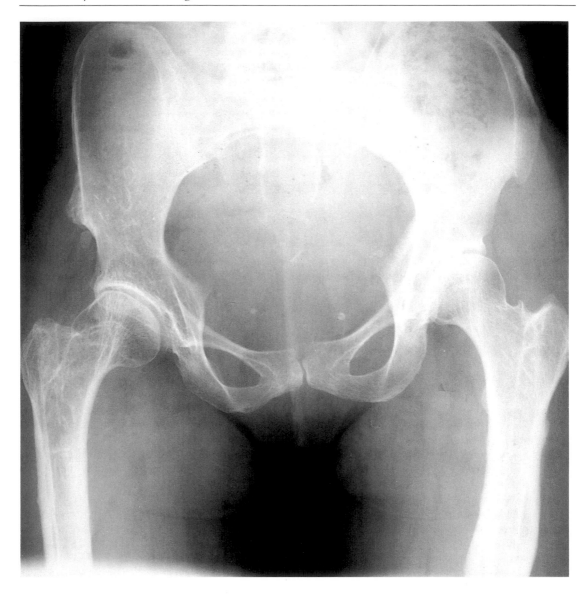

Figure 5.11   Osteogenesis imperfecta. X-ray shows
evidence of previous multiple fractures, with some
deformity of the long bones and protrusio acetabuli.

often with marked callus formation, which may suggest a sarcoma (see Figure 5.11). Generalized osteopenia is common, contributed to partly by the disease and partly by the disuse atrophy caused by limb deformity.

Other investigations

Investigation of the family for evidence of osteogenesis imperfecta may be necessary for genetic counselling. In future this may be simplified by the use of gene probes to identify the specific mutations involved.

Diagnosis

The severe forms of osteogenesis imperfecta are radiologically distinct. Dwarfism is associated with extraordinary limb deformities. Chest wall collapse brings sufferers to hospital with pneumonia and heart failure.

The diagnosis of mild forms depends on the presence of extraskeletal features, such as blue sclerae and family history, which are not constant. The bones are either radiologically normal or suggest generalized osteoporosis. Bone density is reduced. It may be hard to distinguish the mild forms from idiopathic juvenile osteoporosis in the adolescent, although the latter is usually self-limiting. Mild osteogenesis imperfecta in women may first present as postmenopausal osteoporosis[11] and in the absence of the extraskeletal features or a family history of osteogenesis imperfecta or genetic analysis, may never be distinguished from ordinary postmenopausal osteoporosis.

Treatment

The incidence of fracture rises in childhood, falls in adolescence, remains low in men but and rises again in women with the advent of postmenopausal bone loss, when hormone replacement therapy should be considered.[11] Orthopaedic advice is required for fractures and skeletal deformity, as complex problems may arise. Dental surgery and orthodontic care will be needed for those with dental problems. Patients and their families benefit by counselling, and by measures to prevent and treat complications. Children with osteogenesis imperfecta are in the same dilemma as patients with severe osteoporosis. Exercise and mobility must be maintained so as to conserve bone strength and muscle power against the atrophy of disuse, but mobility brings with it the risk of further fractures. Children and adults who are more severely deformed may need the services of a skilled rehabilitation unit to assist mobility and activities of daily life. Adaptations to wheelchairs and car seats, the provision of moulded and padded body shells to cushion spinal deformities, adapted shoes and hearing aids are among the aids to daily living that can be provided.

There is no specific medical treatment and the rarity and variability of the disease will ensure that successful controlled clinical trials of a candidate therapy will be hard to achieve. There are anecdotal reports of improvement from hydroxyapatite compound in children and more recently from bisphosphonates. They might be improving the secondary osteoporosis rather than the underlying disease.

Considerable distress may be caused when a child with osteogenesis imperfecta is brought to hospital with repeated fractures and 'baby battering' is suspected. In so rare a condition skilled medical evidence to refute this may be hard to come by. Wherever a Brittle Bone Society has been set up, as in the UK, to provide counselling, expert advice and to support research, parents should be encouraged to join.

FIBROUS DYSPLASIA

Fibrous dysplasia is a rare disorder characterized by lesions of fibrous tissue within bone. With monostotic involvement, lesions are mainly in the skull, face or ribs. With polyostotic involvement, lesions are found in all bones. The latter may be associated with pigmented cutaneous lesions and precocious puberty (Albright's syndrome).

Epidemiology

This rare condition is not hereditable and affects the sexes equally, although Albright's syndrome, which includes up to one-third of those with polyostotic fibrous dysplasia, is uncommon in males.

Pathophysiology

Sharply demarcated lesions are found in the bone, filled by fibrous tissue which may contain cysts or spicules of woven bone and cartilage. There is also osteoclastic proliferation with bone destruction.

Signs and symptoms

Fibrous dysplasia causes expansion of bone, which is painless unless fractures occur. These lesions, which may be unilateral, happen at any age and lead to deformity. The femur and tibia are the bones most commonly involved. Vertebral body lesions may result in compression fractures and paraplegia. Secondary sarcomatous change has been occasionally reported. Children with Albright's syndrome commonly present with precocious puberty (in girls this is accompanied by vaginal bleeding), and may also present with pain in the leg or a fracture. Cutaneous pigmentation consists of flat, light to dark brown lesions with an irregular border and of variable size. Associated endocrine disorders have included goitre, hyperthyroidism, acromegaly, Cushing's syndrome, accelerated skeletal growth, gynaecomastia and parathyroid enlargement.

Biochemistry

The serum calcium level is normal but the serum phosphate may be low. The serum alkaline phosphatase and urinary hydroxyproline output are sometimes increased, reflecting high bone turnover.

Radiology

Radiolucent areas are seen (Figure 5.12). These may be cystic in the cortex or have a 'ground glass' appearance in the medulla due to the spicules of woven bone. With expansion the bone appears structureless with the loss of the distinction between cortex and medulla. Pathological fractures and deformities are also seen. The appearances usually remain unchanged during adult life.

Diagnosis

These lesions need to be distinguished from those of osteitis fibrosa cystica or osteoclastoma. A normal blood biochemical profile will exclude the former, but bone biopsy is needed to exclude the latter.

Treatment

There is no specific treatment.

HYPOPHOSPHATASIA

Hypophosphatasia is a hereditable disorder seen mainly in infants, in whom the prognosis is poor, although an adult form does occur. Fractures and defective mineralization may be caused by abnormal osteoid being formed by

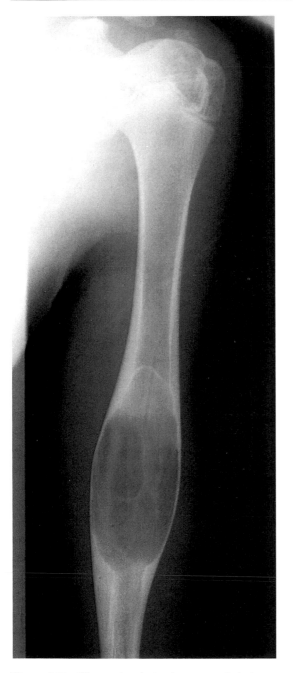

Figure 5.12 Fibrous dysplasia. A monostotic lesion in the humerus.

osteoblasts with secondary loss or reduction of alkaline phosphatase activity. This decreased or absent alkaline phosphatase activity is seen in tissues as well as serum and the amino acid phosphorylethanolamine is found in the plasma and urine. Serum calcium is often elevated, and there may be hypercalciuria, proteinuria and the evidence of impaired renal function. The urinary hydroxyproline output is low.

The whole skeleton is involved, shows defective ossification and is deformed, although occasionally it can appear normal apart from fracture. Symptoms of hypercalcaemia may be present and blue sclerae are often seen. Adults may present with bone pain or fractures and on investigation there is mild osteoporosis associated with low serum alkaline phosphatase and detectable urinary phosphorylethanolamine.

Low alkaline phosphatase levels are also found in scurvy, severe malnutrition, hypothyroidism and idiopathic hypercalcaemia. The presence of phosphorylethanolamine in the urine is also not specific and found in liver disease, scurvy, erythroblastosis, coeliac disease and occasionally in normal adults.

There is no satisfactory treatment.

OSTEOMYELITIS

Osteomyelitis is still an important cause of bone pain, particularly of the spine, although it is not as common as in the past. Some patients develop osteomyelitis as a complication of AIDS. Osteomyelitis has a high morbidity, significant mortality and outcome is related to delay in diagnosis. It must not be forgotten.

In adults, osteomyelitis of long bones is most commonly a complication of prosthetic joint surgery, but osteomyelitis of the vertebrae is usually by haematogenous spread. *Staphylococcus aureus* is the commonest infective agent (and anti-staphylolysin titres may be

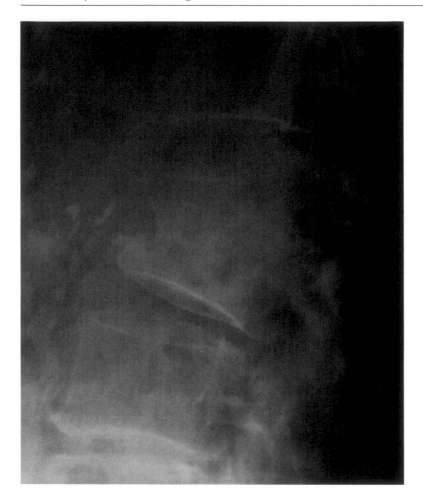

Figure 5.13 Osteomyelitis affecting two adjacent vertebrae with rapid destruction of bone and disc. The cortex is destroyed in contrast to osteoporotic vertebral collapse.

helpful), but Gram-negative bacilli and mycobacteria are also important causes. The source is often the skin or urinary tract.

Infection of the vertebral body readily spreads and it is not uncommon for two adjacent vertebrae to become involved. Central spread may result in spinal cord compression, and paraspinal spread in the lumbar region can produce the classic psoas abscess. Spread can also result in retropharyngeal abscesses, mediastinitis, empyema, pericarditis or peritonitis.

Most patients have fever, back pain with local tenderness and muscle spasm, but the elderly or those on glucocorticoids do not always show a normal inflammatory response to infection. Sometimes a source of infection is obvious, but there is a danger that loin pain and fever following cystitis may be interpreted as pyelonephritis without due consideration of the possibility of haematogenous spread to a lumbar vertebra.

Fever, weight loss and elevation of erythrocyte sedimentation rate, plasma viscosity and C-reactive protein serve to distinguish spinal osteomyelitis from osteoporotic vertebral collapse. Blood cultures may identify the organism but aspiration or surgical exploration may be necessary.

Radiology shows the rapid destruction of vertebral bone and disc (see Figure 5.13), and CT scanning may detect the formation of any soft tissue abscesses. Radioisotope scanning with ^{99m}Tc is not so helpful as it lacks specificity. Gallium-67 is more informative.

Treatment is with appropriate antibiotics, usually for six weeks or more.

MUSCULOSKELETAL PAIN RESEMBLING BONE PAIN

Polymyalgia rheumatica, hypothyroidism and dyskinetic Parkinsonism may all cause diffuse musculoskeletal pain. Polymyalgia rheumatica is characterized by marked stiffness after rest, an elevated sedimentation rate or plasma viscosity with a rapid and often dramatic response to glucocorticoid therapy. Hypothyroidism is detected by clinical history, delayed reflex recovery time and thyroid function tests, and Parkinsonism by the clinical features of the disease and by improvement with levodopa therapy. Bone pain is characteristically increased at night and unaffected by joint movement. Differentiation of bone pain from these other causes of pain is thus possible on the clinical history. Light percussion over superficial bones (sternum, pelvic rim, medial aspect of the tibia) may elicit tenderness in diffuse bone pain, but not in other causes of diffuse pain.

PRACTICAL POINTS

- Other causes of osteopenia, fracture and bone pain must be considered before diagnosing osteoporosis.

- A combination of vitamin D depletion and mild secondary hyperparathyroidism is common in housebound or institutionalized elderly people, and may present as osteoporosis.

- Overt osteomalacia is also seen in the elderly, occasionally in those who fracture the proximal femur. It is readily treatable and can be diagnosed biochemically, but more reliably by bone biopsy.

- Bone pain and pathological fractures that are due to malignancy or osteomyelitis must be excluded.

- Paget's disease and hyperparathyroidism cause bone pain.

- Osteogenesis imperfecta, a rare group of hereditable disorders, is associated with bone fragility and presents with fractures—usually in childhood.

REFERENCES

1. Peacock M. Osteomalacia and rickets. In: Nordin BEC ed. *Metabolic bone and stone disease*, 2nd Edition. Churchill Livingstone: Edinburgh (1984), pp. 71–111.

2. Fraser D. Vitamin D. *Lancet* (1995), **345**: 104–7.

3. Wilkins WE, Chalmers A, Sanerkin NG et al. Osteomalacia in the elderly: the value of radio-isotope bone scanning in patients with equivocal biochemistry. *Age Ageing* (1983), **12**: 195–200.

4. Mundy GR, Ibbotson KJ, D'Souza SM et al. The hypercalcemia of cancer. Clinical implications and pathogenic mechanisms. *N Engl J Med* (1984), **311**: 47–9.

5. Munday GR, Martin TJ. The hypercalcemia of malignancy: pathogenesis and management. *Metabolism* (1982), **31**: 1247–77.

6. Roodman GD. Current hypothesis for the etiology of Paget's disease. In: Kohler P. ed. *Current opinion in endocrinology and diabetes, Volume 1. Parathyroid and calcium and mineral disorders*. Current Science Group US: Philadelphia (1984).

7. Diamond T, Ng ATM, Levy S et al. Estrogen replacement may be an alternative to parathyroid surgery for the treatment of osteoporosis in older postmenopausal women presenting with primary hyperparathyroidism: a preliminary report. *Osteoporos Int* (1996), **6**: 329–33.

8. Smith R, Francis MJO, Houghton GR. *The brittle bone syndrome: osteogenesis imperfecta*. Butterworths: London (1983).

9. Byers PH. Disorders of collagen biosynthesis and structure. In: Scriver CR, Beaudet AL, Sly WS et al. eds. *The metabolic and molecular basis of inherited disease*. 7th Edition. New York: McGraw Hill (1995), pp. 4029–77.

10. Sillence DO, Senn A, Danks DM. Genetic heterogeneity in osteogenesis imperfecta. *J Med Genet* (1979), **16**: 101–16.

11. Paterson CR, McAllion S, Stellman JL. Osteogenesis imperfecta after the menopause. *N Engl J Med* (1984), **310**: 1694–6.

6   Fractures in osteoporosis

THE FRACTURE SUFFERER

Old bones break easily and age is the strongest determinant of bone weakness. The two most important sites of osteoporosis-related fracture are the hip and the spine. At the age of 50, a woman of European stock has an approximately two out of five lifetime risk of sustaining a hip fracture. That still means that three out of five women will escape and raises the question of who is the woman most likely to fracture? Epidemiologists have looked at numerous associated and lifestyle factors in longitudinal and cross-sectional studies of populations.[1,2] As a woman grows older, these factors become more predictive of fracture, particularly fracture of the hip. A profile can now be constructed.

She will be in her seventh decade or older. She will have had a previous low impact fracture such as a Colles',[3] an X-ray will show compression deformities of several vertebral bodies[4,5] and she will be in the lowest quartile for her age group for femoral neck bone density measured by DXA and calcaneal bone density measured by ultrasound.[6] Her mother also will have had a low impact fracture.[7] She will have lead a generally sedentary life, had few or no children and had an early artificial or natural menopause and not taken HRT. She will have a white skin[8] and be more likely to derive from northern than southern European stock.[9] She will eat meat rather than being a vegetarian, will be a smoker, a coffee-lover and a more than moderate alcohol-drinker.[10] She will be frail rather than robust, living in an institution rather than in her own home and will have a low body mass index, weak strength of grip, weak quadriceps muscles and inability to stand up from a chair without using her hands. Once on her feet she will show increased body sway.[11] If she does live at home, efforts to save her from fractures by removing domestic hazards will have been of no avail,[12] but if she is lucky enough to be wearing impact-absorbing hip protector pads when she falls, she will almost certainly escape a hip fracture.[13]

The man most likely to get a hip fracture will also be elderly, frail rather than robust, will have a low femoral neck bone density and will be a meat-eater and a more than moderate alcohol-drinker, but whether or not he is/had been a smoker and whether or not other members of his family had osteoporosis, will be less relevant.

In either sex some contributory illness, such as arthritis, stroke, dementia or poor eyesight is likely to be present.

Age-related loss of bone mass is paralleled by age-related increases in fractures of the distal radius, proximal humerus, femoral neck and vertebral bodies. Whereas osteoporotic fractures of the vertebral bodies may occur spontaneously and sometimes without pain, osteoporotic fractures of the long bones are usually precipitated by a fall and are painful. What would seem a trivial fall may result in fracture, and most occur from standing height or less. Such falls are common in the elderly (see Chapter 2).

VERTEBRAL FRACTURES

One in three vertebral fractures present with sudden onset of back pain. The remaining two-thirds of patients have chronic spinal shrinkage identified when X-rayed for chronic back pain, loss of height or stoop.

The acute vertebral crush fracture syndrome (AVCFS)

Clinical features

The most commonly affected vertebrae are from T8 to L3, with the first crush affecting T12. The dominant symptom is pain, which is felt diffusely in the back, is related to movement and reduced or abolished by rest. It is often referred around the body, usually symmetrically. When this occurs, pain reliably follows the dermatomes so a fracture of T9 gives rise to pain felt not only in the back but also anteriorly at rib margin level, a fracture at T11 causes pain felt in the abdomen at the level of the umbilicus, a fracture of L1 is referred down to the groin and a fracture of L3 to the anterior thighs and knees. These are sometimes described as band-like or belt-like pains but, on careful analysis, they are found to consist of disconnected patches of pain relating to the anterior and posterior primary rami of the corresponding nerve roots. The acute episode may be so painful that it is accompanied by shock, pallor and vomiting, the latter being exceedingly painful itself, as is

sneezing or coughing in subjects with both respiratory disease and vertebral crush fracture.

The severe pain of a crush fracture generally subsides within a week or two with bed-rest, but further crushing of the same vertebral body or fractures of adjacent ones may lead to a repetition of the original episode. It is unusual for an osteoporotic individual to complain of severe unrelenting pain which does not improve to a more bearable level after about three weeks. Persistence of severe pain beyond three weeks suggests that other causes such as infection, cancer or myelomatosis should be sought. Despite this, it has to be recognized that some osteoporosis sufferers complain of severe and enduring back pain, unrelieved even by opiate analgesics. Sometimes this is interpreted as a 'cry for help' by a lonely and disabled elderly person. Against this, an osteoporosis sufferer complained of enduring pain which led her twice to make suicide attempts although she was well looked after by a devoted husband.

The mechanism for chronic pain associated with spinal shrinkage tendered by the postmortem studies of Hoyland et al.[14] needs to be remembered. This is that otherwise unexplained back pain can be associated with compression of the veins which run through the intervertebral foramina, resulting in oedema, congestion and fibrosis of nerve roots distal to the compression.[14]

AVCFS frequently occurs in elderly women already known to be at risk through chronic disease such as rheumatoid arthritis or who are receiving treatment with corticosteroids. Men are also affected (see Figure 6.1). A vertebral crush fracture is a pernicious complication for about one in four patients receiving heart or liver transplants and is often the first intimation of the rare pregnancy-associated osteoporosis. Sometimes these underlying causes are present as part of the clinical picture and may dominate it to the point where the osteoporotic fracture is not immediately recognizable. A spinal fracture in a woman with

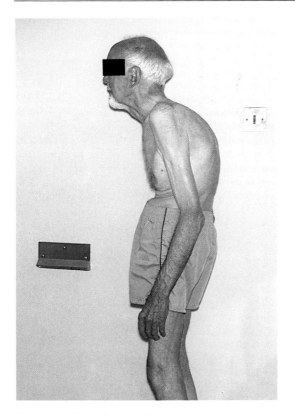

Figure 6.1 This 70-year-old man presented with a three-year history of pain in his back, but there had been no sudden or severe episodes. Bone biopsy showed osteoporosis.

able variation between individuals as to the bone weakening effects of glucocorticoids. In some patients a vertebral crush fracture may occur within a year of starting treatment while others seem to be resistant. This resistance may reflect either a high initial peak bone mass or an increased ability to inactivate the hormone in the liver.

Physical signs of AVCFS

The physical signs of AVCFS include stiffness and rigidity of movement caused by protective muscle spasm, seen and felt as stiffening and contraction of the paraspinal muscles symmetrically. All spinal movements are grossly restricted. Gentle percussion with a soft-nosed patella hammer over the spinous processes may localize precisely the site of the fracture. With severe pain there is often radiation up and down the spine to neighbouring dermatomes, both in subjective pain and in elicited tenderness. Significant negatives are the absence of signs of neurological disturbance and a normal straight-leg raising test (provided that this can be done without moving the affected part of the spine, and thus increasing local pain). However, rare instances of spinal cord pressure in men with osteoporotic dorsal spinal fractures have been recorded.[16]

rheumatoid arthritis may easily be missed because of the pain on movement of other parts of the body. Fragility fractures are not rare in advanced ankylosing spondylitis, usually in men,[15] who are in danger of being treated as having a local recurrence or exacerbation of the underlying spinal disease. Despite this, every doctor who is interested in osteoporosis will have met individuals who present with loss of height, even as much as 200 mm, yet who have noticed little or no pain although an X-ray shows collapse of several vertebral bodies. There is also very consider-

Investigations

The X-rays will show wedging and collapse of the affected vertebra but in the early stages it may be difficult to tell whether the more obvious radiological changes are in fact the cause of the current symptoms, particularly where previous episodes of crush fracture have occurred. Localization must depend on the clinical picture unless a previous X-ray is available showing which changes were previously present and which are new. After several

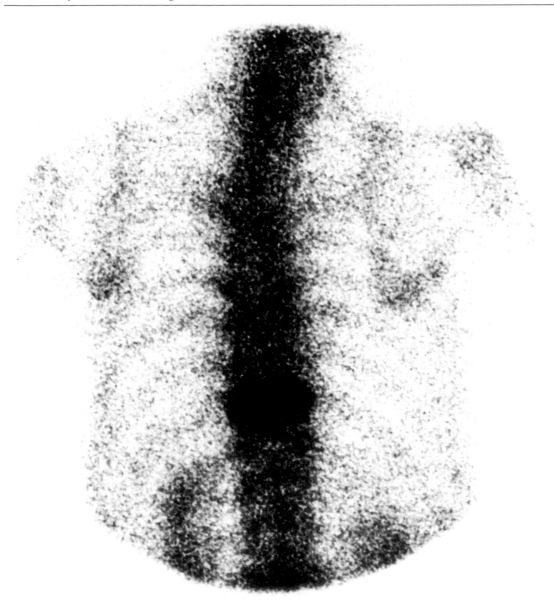

Figure 6.2   Radioisotope bone scan showing
increased tracer uptake in a recently collapsed
osteoporotic vertebra.

days (seldom less than a week), there is evidence of internal callus formation, with the vertebra becoming more dense. Only rarely is there evidence of a callus outside the affected vertebral body, presumably reflecting the occurrence of an extra-osseous haematoma. The X-rays will also show osteoporosis in neighbouring vertebrae, making other causes of collapse fracture, such as invasion of the bone by metastatic tumour or osteolytic Paget's disease, less likely.

The radioisotope bone scan is helpful as it will localize fairly precisely the most recent site of fracture (see Figure 6.2), and differentiate from metastatic disease—in which multiple 'hot spots' can usually be seen. Blood tests show no changes at first but after a few days the plasma viscosity and erythrocyte sedimentation rate will rise slightly as part of the acute phase reaction and the plasma alkaline phosphatase will rise in response to the bone disturbance caused by the fracture. They may be more useful in excluding other causes such as metastases or myeloma. Breath hydrogen tests have been used to detect lactose intolerance and other forms of malabsorption.

Mrs M B, aged 65 years, developed rheumatoid arthritis at the age of 62 years. Pain and swelling failed to respond to nonsteroidal anti-inflammatory drugs. When she was 65, her doctor had put her on prednisolone treatment, 5 mg twice daily, with immediate symptomatic benefit, greater mobility and gain in weight. However, 11 months later she developed acute back pain and examination showed crush fractures of T11 and T12. After two weeks in hospital, treated with a short course of calcitonin, reduction of corticosteroid dosage, and bed-rest followed by gentle mobilization in the hydrotherapy pool, she became pain-free and was able to return home. She was commenced on cyclical etidronate to prevent further bone loss and reduce risk of fracture.

Acute vertebral collapse

Differential diagnosis

The pain of acute vertebral collapse fracture must be distinguished from that of vertebral collapse secondary to osteolytic malignant deposits, Paget's disease, and especially myelomatosis. Less common are infections of a vertebra by staphylococcus, typhoid or tuberculosis. In the lower lumbar vertebrae, prolapsed intervertebral disc does not often pose a diagnostic problem because it generally affects a younger age group and symptoms are one-sided. Cachexia suggests malignancy or infection. Helpful investigations include vertebral body biopsy or aspiration (which is usually done under radiological guidance) or computerized axial tomography or magnetic resonance imaging, which may reveal a paraspinal soft tissue mass when there is an abscess or neoplastic growth. The bone isoenzyme of plasma alkaline phosphatase will be considerably elevated in Paget's disease, less so in other bone conditions. Fever, a marked acute phase response, blood and urine culture, and anti-staphylolysin titre are all helpful in the diagnosis of infections. Serum immunoelectrophoresis and examination for light chains in the urine (Bence–Jones proteinuria) are part of the screening for myelomatosis.

Treatment of acute vertebral collapse

The acute vertebral collapse fracture is often so painful that the patient *must* rest; the only comfortable position may be supine in bed with one or two pillows. Some patients are able to rest in a chair, which is useful in older patients who have respiratory problems when lying flat. Pain is best managed by simple analgesics such as paracetamol (acetaminophen) or coproxamol. However, nonsteroidal anti-inflammatory drugs or even opiates may be needed on occasion as adequate pain control is essential. It is useful to potentiate the effects of analgesics by concurrent use of an anxiolytic such as diazepam. The latter are sold as central muscle relaxants but it is doubtful whether they have this mode of action faced with the intense spasm of the spinal muscles seen in this condition. Peripheral muscle relaxants such as methocarbamol are of no value. Concurrent corticosteroid therapy should not be reduced or stopped in the acute phase so as not to precipitate adrenal insufficiency. Reduction of corticosteroid dose can start at a later date. Calcitonin by subcutaneous or intramuscular injection or nasal insufflation has an analgesic effect on spinal pain.

Of physical measures, few are of much help. Some patients feel better with heat, such as a hot water bottle, on the affected area. Careful positioning of pillows may be essential for patients with concurrent respiratory difficulties. There is no specific recommended duration for bed-rest; it should be the minimum that the patient can manage as immobility will lead to bone loss but more importantly it will make rehabilitation more difficult and prolonged. Early X-ray of the spine is not essential and, like mobilization, it should not be undertaken until there is adequate pain control.

During the immediate convalescent phase it is the authors' practice to give salmon calcitonin 100 IU subcutaneously daily for 21 days if pain is severe, based on its known relief of pain in this condition. Spinal braces should be avoided, as they are only rarely necessary for those patients whose osteoporosis is so severe that almost all the lower thoracic and lumbar vertebrae are affected and deformed. Braces are poorly tolerated and further restrict the movement on which maintenance of adequate bone density depends.

Finally, treatment should be considered to reduce the risk of further osteoporotic-related fractures (see Chapter 9).

Complications of vertebral collapse

In thoracic crush fracture the pain may lead to breathing difficulty and broncho-pneumonia from failure to clear the lung bases. Should collapse and hypotension occur following too early withdrawal of glucocorticoid treatment (see above), 100 mg of hydrocortisone sodium succinate should be given intravenously. If there has been any doubt, the rapid improvement brought about by intravenous glucocorticoids in patients with adrenal insufficiency is diagnostic. Transient hypercalcaemia and hypercalciuria commonly follow fracture and on occasions may be associated with renal stone formation.

Complications of chronic spinal shrinkage

Many patients with vertebral osteoporosis just lose height without the typical episodes of acute pain that can be associated with vertebral collapse. They then present with complications of chronic spinal shrinkage.

Neck problems

As the individual loses height and kyphosis increases, secondary 'postural' pains become dominant. Thus, the complaint of a stiff painful neck and of tension headache is common in the elderly woman as she tries to hold up her head by hyperextending the neck. Neck pain can at first be relieved by sitting down in an easy chair and allowing the head to fall back but even this becomes difficult in time as dorsal kyphosis increases. Easy chairs are designed for people with normal backs and the rake of the seat back soon becomes insufficient to support the head without undue effort by the cervical extensor muscles. At this stage the osteoporotic elderly woman shares certain problems with younger men or women who have advanced ankylosing spondylitis. For example, they can sit, watch television, enjoy theatre or drive a car, but cannot drink from a glass while standing up and have

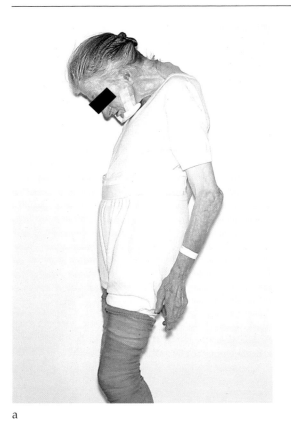

a

increasing difficulty in crossing a road because of loss of upward gaze (see Figure 6.3).

At a later stage still, the splenius capitis muscle and other cervical extensor muscles seem to 'give up' and there follows a phase which has been called 'toggle neck'—the head can just be kept up if lifted passively but will fall to a flexed position, chin on chest, if the patient looks down. Finally, the chin rests permanently on the chest, a condition which makes anaesthetization for intercurrent surgical emergencies hazardous because of the extreme difficulty in intubation.

At a more mundane level, the sufferer experiences difficulties in getting clothing to fit, while such day-to-day problems as obtaining a comfortable chair can also make life more miserable than it need be. Individually moulded and padded body shells may allow for a comfortable sedentary life when there is advanced kyphosis.

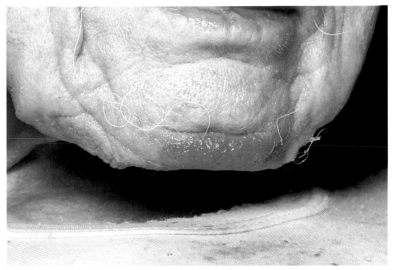

b

Figure 6.3 (a) A 78-year-old woman with advanced osteoporosis. She is unable to look ahead, but attempts to do so by flexing her knees. (b) Her chin is in constant contact with her sternum resulting in soreness of the skin.

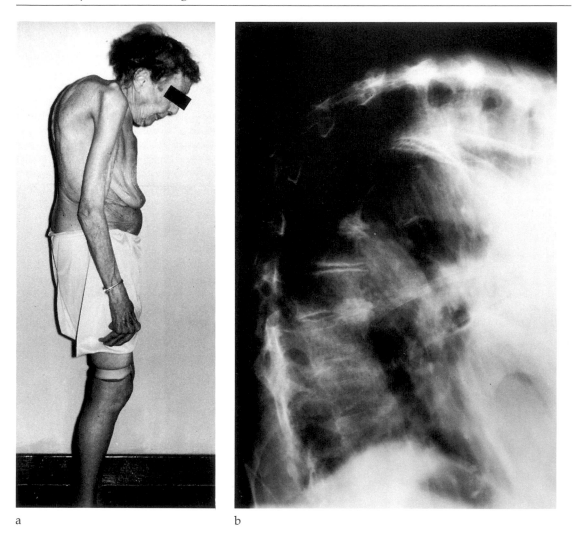

a   b

Figure 6.4   (a,b) Severe spinal osteoporosis in a
woman with longstanding but mild rheumatoid
arthritis. She has a protuberant abdomen and suffers
from reflux oesophagitis.

Difficulty in upward gaze may require the
use of prism spectacles and, fortunately, light-
weight prism glasses made with fresnel lenses
are now obtainable. Some of the problems of
the patient with advanced osteoporosis are
illustrated in Figure 6.4.

Decreased lung and abdominal capacity

As the spine shrinks the space in the two
primary coelomic cavities, thorax and
abdomen, is reduced and changes shape. The

chest, on postero-anterior X-ray, is compressed laterally, the lung fields are small with high diaphragms and the ribs appear crowded. On lateral X-ray, the postero-anterior diameter of the thorax is greatly increased. In some elderly sufferers, particularly where some degree of osteomalacia coexists, the sternum and the manubrium remodel to a 'Z' shape with a decreased angle between the manubrium and the sternum, and below this the sternum is bowed outwards by the pressure of the abdominal contents (see Figure 6.5). Lung capacity is reduced and with it the ability to overcome coexisting lung disease, particularly asthma, bronchitis and emphysema. Bronchial pneumonia presents special hazards in those with advanced osteoporosis. Excessive coughing and the use of physiotherapy percussion on the chest to help clear sputum carry the danger of fracture of the fragile ribs.

The abdominal cavity is similarly constrained. The woman who is body-conscious commonly first notices the protrusion of the anterior abdominal wall and may think that she is getting fatter when in fact her weight is steady or falling. Some women will resort to wearing elasticated corselettes hoping that these will make them slimmer, but these may only lead to breathlessness on exertion by restricting diaphragmatic movement. The shrinkage of the lower thoracic and lumbar segments means that the woman will show increased abdominal transverse creases and a finger placed between the tenth rib and the iliac crest will show that this space, normally 5 cm or more in height, is reduced even to the point of painful impaction of the ribs on the pelvic brim. In some women with narrow chests and wide pelves the thorax may descend within the pelvis (see Figure 6.6). In others, particularly if there is some scoliosis, only one side will impact, the other remaining clear. Intertrigo of the transverse skin folds over the abdomen may occur. These moist areas become colonized by yeasts and other commensals, causing soreness, desquamation and the production of a typical unpleasant cheesy odour (see Figure 6.7). Careful atten-

tion to hygiene and drying with toilet powder, together with the occasional use of antifungal ('athlete's foot') preparations which can keep the area sanitary, may be necessary. An anteroposterior X-ray of the abdomen may reveal that the domes of the diaphragm reach up to the level of the posterior part of the third ribs and it is this, together with the loss of space in the thorax, which leads to breathlessness on exertion compounded by tight garments around the waist if these are worn.

There are two further consequences of decreased abdominal capacity. One, which is common, is hiatus hernia, with the typical symptoms of acid reflux on lying down or stooping forward. The other, less common, and perhaps related more to an associated collagen weakness, is pelvic floor prolapse, either rectal, uterine or both. However, stress incontinence does not seem to be more frequent in osteoporotic subjects than in others of the same age.

X-rays of the abdomen or lumbar spine often reveal marked calcification of the aorta in contrast to the lack of calcium in the spine (see Figure 6.8). It is not known why calcium is lost from some sites but deposited in others.

OSTEOPOROTIC FRACTURES OTHER THAN OF THE SPINE

Osteoporotic fractures of long bones do not differ from fractures in normal bones, except in the degree of trauma needed to produce them, nor do they differ as far as immediate treatment is concerned. A fracture is dramatic. It follows trauma and the limb and the patient are immediately disabled. The diagnosis is made on clinical grounds, supported by appropriate X-rays. Treatment of an osteoporosis-related long bone fracture follows the usual well-known principles of fracture management: namely, correction of deformity and fixation of the bone in the corrected position until union has occurred, which takes

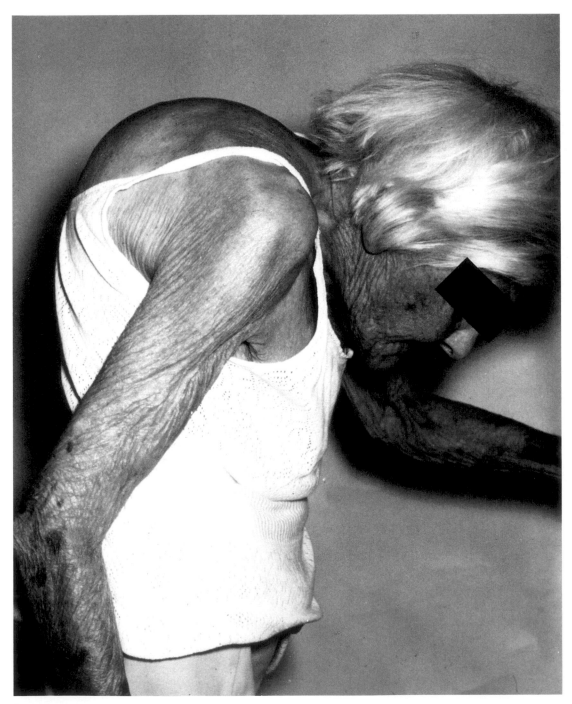

a

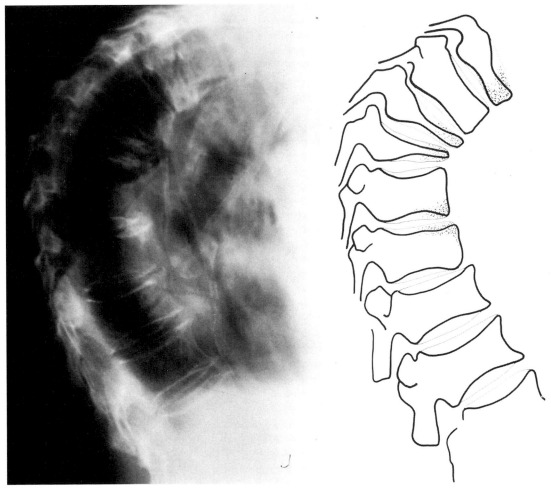

b

Figure 6.5   (a) An elderly spinster with longstanding rheumatoid arthritis. X-rays (b) show extreme dorsal kyphosis and (c) zigzag deformity of the sternum. Postmortem examination showed both osteoporosis and osteomalacia.

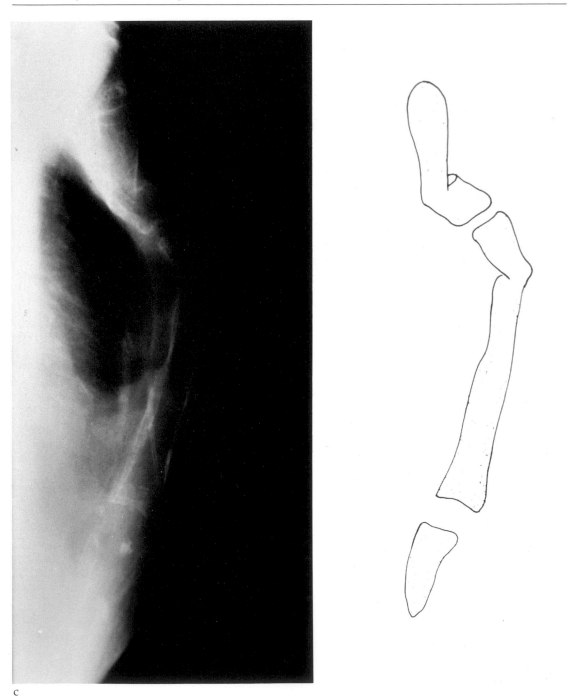

c

Figure 6.5 *continued*

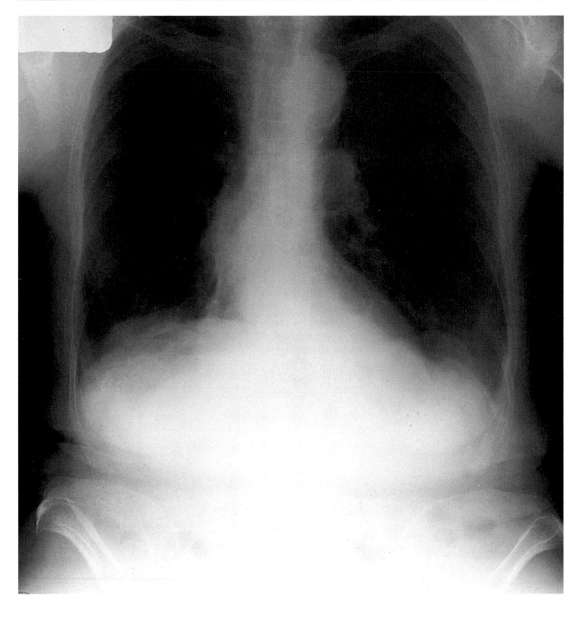

Figure 6.6   The lower ribs abut on the pelvic brim causing local pain and worsening of the breathlessness of this woman with chronic obstructive airways disease. She was also concerned about her protuberant abdomen, but could not tolerate a girdle.

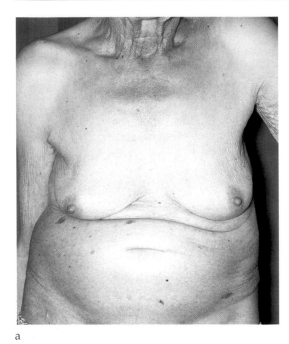

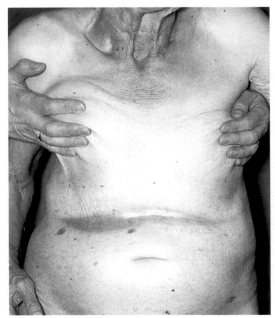

a   b

Figure 6.7   (a) Abdominal creases and (b) intertrigo.

place within a normal period of time in osteo-porotic bone.

Unfortunately, the casualty officer, fracture clinic or general practitioner may not perceive the contribution of the underlying bone weakness, and lose a valuable opportunity for secondary prevention. Elderly patients with fractures should be assessed for causes of fracture and given advice and treatment to reduce risk of further fracture when the immediate problems of the fracture have been dealt with. Indeed, the bone weakness may be only one of several contributory causes that should be considered: poor eyesight, locomo-tor difficulties from arthritis or stroke, tempo-rary disturbances of consciousness as in Adams–Stokes attacks. (For further discussion, see Chapter 2.)

Fractures of ribs

Rib fractures (see Figure 6.9) may complicate other fractures in elderly subjects who fall. Sometimes they are only evident when callus is seen on a later X-ray of the chest or if a radioisotope bone scan is performed. Spontaneous rib fractures are an early feature of Cushing's syndrome, often present when

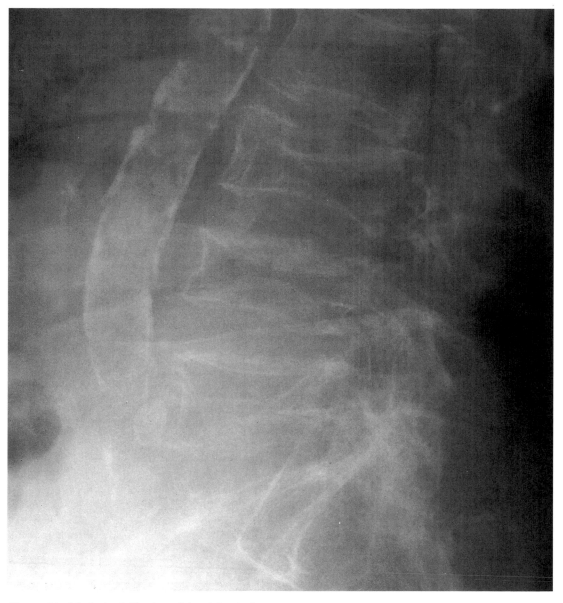

Figure 6.8 Marked calcification of the abdominal
aorta and osteoporosis of the lumbar spine.

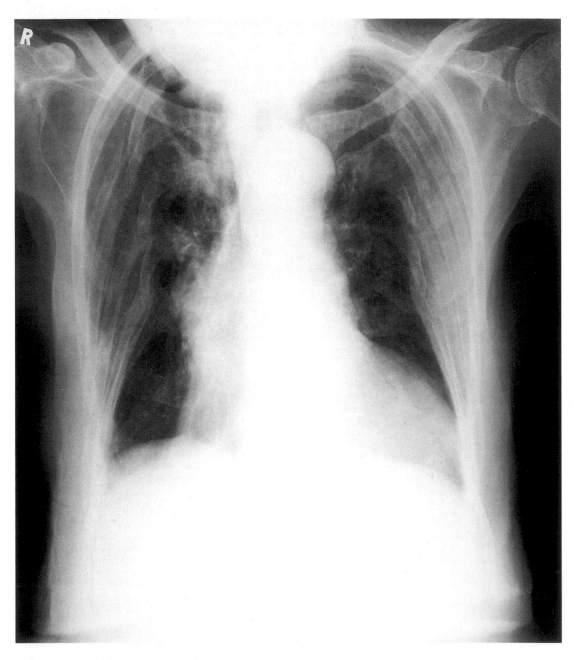

Figure 6.9   Marked osteoporosis and multiple fractures of the ribs associated with rheumatoid arthritis and glucocorticoid therapy.

the diagnosis is first made. When accompanying more serious fractures, such as of the hip, they increase the likelihood of respiratory complications. Conversely, coughing can cause a rib fracture in osteoporotic subjects, and be mistaken for pleurisy.

Fractures of the wrist

These are generally caused by falls on the outstretched hand (see Figure 2.3c). Not all wrist fractures present with the classical 'dinner fork' deformity of a Colles' fracture. A hairline fracture without displacement is not infrequent in osteoporosis and can be difficult to see on X-ray until a few days have elapsed. Moreover, the fracture may have impacted and stabilized itself, thus minimizing deformity and permitting some use of the hand. Hairline fractures of the wrist can easily be confused with arthritis of the wrist, particularly in subjects who already have arthritis elsewhere.

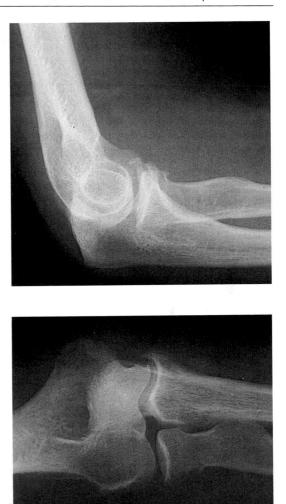

Figure 6.10 Fracture of the neck of the radius.

A 54-year-old woman suffering from rheumatoid arthritis was admitted to the medical ward of a general hospital for intercurrent pneumonia. The right wrist swelled and was correctly diagnosed as a flare of arthritis. Then the left wrist became painful and the same diagnosis was made. As she was by now considerably disabled in dressing and washing, a rheumatological consultation was arranged and it was pointed out that the left wrist had sustained a hairline fracture following a minor fall. Active physiotherapy was obviously inappropriate and a splint was applied.

Persistent pain after a wrist fracture may indicate the onset of algodystrophy and the development of regional osteoporosis (see Chapter 4). Carpal tunnel syndrome is sometimes a late complication of wrist fracture, particularly if there has been difficulty in obtaining a correct reduction of the fracture.

Fracture of the elbow

The commonest osteoporosis-related fracture at the elbow is an impacted subcapital fracture

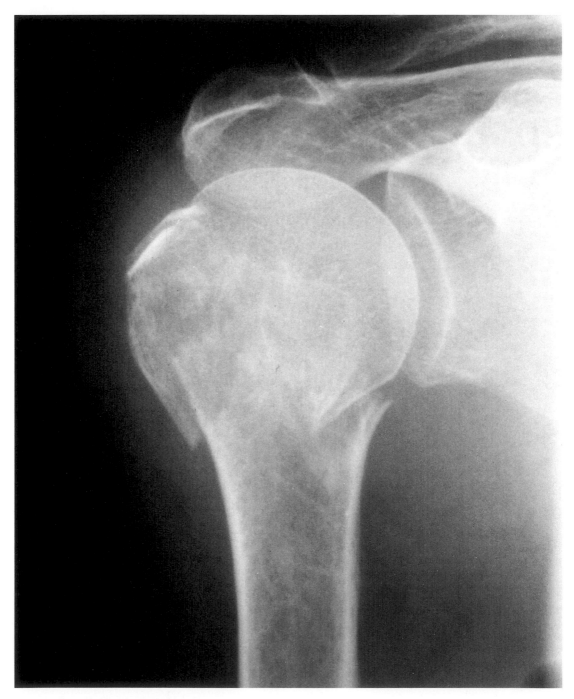

Figure 6.11 Fracture of the proximal humerus.

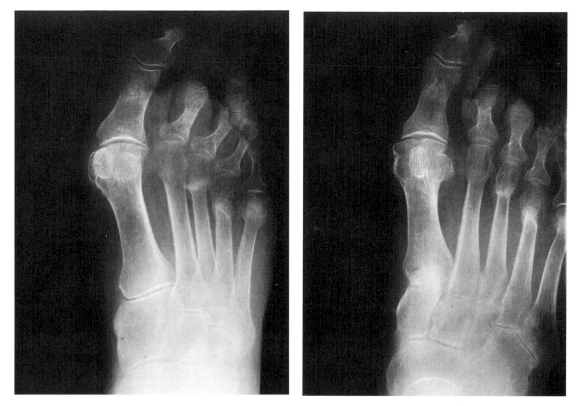

Figure 6.12 March fractures of the metacarpi.

of the radius, usually following a fall on the outstretched hand (see Figure 6.10). The joint remains movable but is painful, and clinically the resemblance to arthritis of the elbow can be close. However, the history of trauma and sometimes the degree of bruising should alert suspicion and the X-ray is of course diagnostic. Treatment is with rest in a sling.

Fracture at the shoulder

This is the third most frequently seen fracture to follow a fall on the outstretched arm.

A 70-year-old woman fell in the garden; as a result she suffered an impacted fracture of the anatomical neck of the right humerus (see Figure 6.11). She had generalized osteopenia. Risk factors for osteoporosis were heavy smoking, chronic obstructive airways disease and recurrent chest infections, in addition to being postmenopausal. Risk factors for falling were living alone, being blind in one eye and having a mild tardive dyskinesia.

Pain and bruising are severe but some movement at the shoulder joint may be retained and impaction of the fragments may stabilize them. It is seldom possible to reduce the fracture at the surgical neck of the humerus without surgery and this is generally not considered worthwhile as the functional results of allowing the fragments to unite in the position they are in are usually quite reasonable. Treatment is with rest in a sling.

Fracture dislocations, which are less common in osteoporotic people, are a different matter and may need surgical reduction.

Fracture of the metatarsal bones (march fracture)

This, and fractures of the ribs, occurs spontaneously in the osteoporosis of Cushing's syndrome and occasionally in other kinds of osteoporosis (see Figure 6.12). They also occur in osteomalacia.

Fracture of the ankle

In rheumatoid arthritis when there is a valgus deformity at the subtaloid joint, there is an increasing valgus strain on the ankle mortise. It is not uncommon, if the patient is osteoporotic, for a stress fracture of the fibula to develop (see Figure 6.13). Again, confusion with an exacerbation of arthritis may occur. The pencil-rolling test is helpful here: a pencil is rolled slowly down the subcutaneous part of the fibula, pressing against the bone. Sharply localized tenderness at the stress fracture line can be detected even before the X-ray becomes diagnostic.

Fractures of the knee

Osteoporotic crush fractures may occur in one or other tibial condyle, usually the lateral tibial condyle. Rarely they occur in the absence of

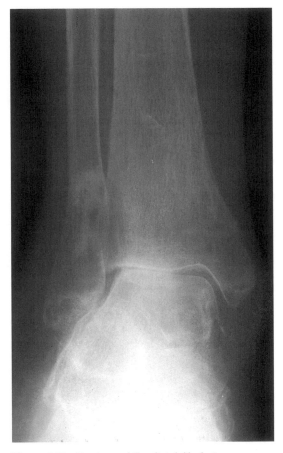

Figure 6.13 Fracture of the distal fibula in a woman with longstanding rheumatoid arthritis and valgus knees and ankles.

inflammatory arthritis of the knee, but usually arthritis is present which has caused both local as well as general osteoporosis. Often some degree of valgus deformity at the knee has already occurred from destruction of the articular cartilage and meniscus. When the patient attempts to walk with the knee in valgus, there is a shift of the compression forces on to the lateral compartment. A crushed tibial condyle may need to be treated by osteotomy or a combination of osteotomy and replacement arthroplasty.

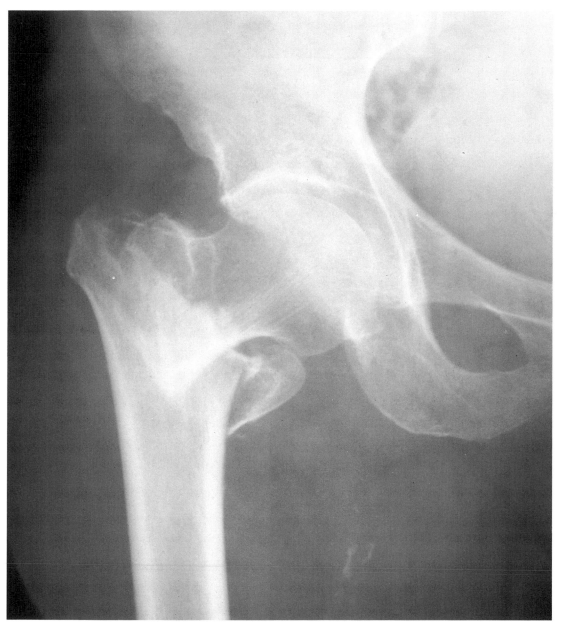

a

Figure 6.14 Fractures of the proximal femur (a) intertrochanteric, and (b) impacted right subcapital.

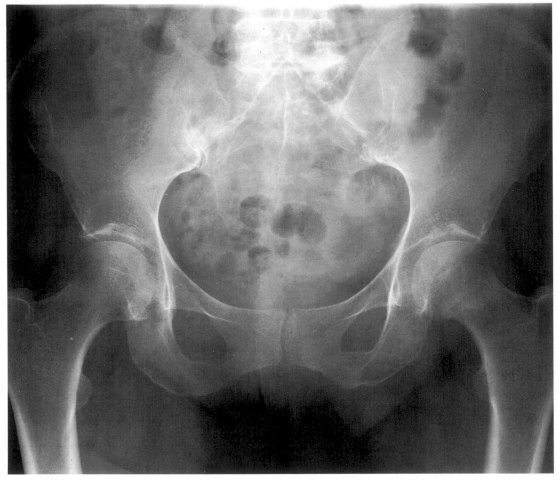

b

Figure 6.14 *continued*

Hip fractures are either transcervical or intertrochanteric (see Figure 6.14) They are negatively associated with osteoarthritis of the hip joint but may complicate inflammatory arthritis. Intertrochanteric and spiral fractures are more frequent in the frail elderly, in those on a poor diet and those with serious inter-current chronic disease. Treatment is by pinning or by total hip replacement arthro-plasty because of the shorter convalescence and decreased mortality. But even so, mortal-ity is still considerable. At the time of the trauma the patient may fall to the ground, lie there unable to get up and may not be discov-ered for many hours if living alone. The following travails include the ambulance ride to hospital, queuing in the casualty and radiology departments, lying on a hard hospital trolley, sometimes for hours, before transfer to a ward where preoperative assessment and eventual operation are awaited. All these delays are unfavourable to survival. Bronchopneumonia and bedsores are common complications. Mortality seems to depend more on the hospital of treatment than the patient. Todd et al.[17] noted differences in 90-day mortality of from 5% to 24% depending on which hospital the patient was taken to.

Many factors contribute to a better outcome. Some of these are organizational, such as maintaining a dedicated hip fracture team and reserving operating theatre time. Very considerable improvements in morbidity and requirements for hospital stay have followed intraoperative intravascular loading to optimal stroke volume monitored by oesophageal Doppler ultrasonography.[18] Others are pharmaceutical, notably prophylaxis against deep vein thrombosis and infection. Early mobilization through a specialist geriatric rehabilitation unit during convalescence is also important. Not only can postoperative mortality be reduced but the proportion of survivors who return to independent living rather than institutional care can be increased.

Stress fractures of the pubic rami

These are more frequent when osteoporosis is complicated by coexisting osteomalacia. Such stress fractures can be difficult to detect on X-ray until time has elapsed and the fracture line subsequently becomes more evident.

Other fractures

This list is by no means exclusive. Fractures of talus, supracondylar fractures of the femur, or of vertebral transverse processes could be added, and indeed fracture of any bone if osteoporosis is severe enough.

Nevertheless, the severe fractures with displacement, the transverse fractures of the tibia, femur or arm and clavicle, or fractures of the skull which are seen in younger people following road traffic accidents and sports injuries are rare in elderly and osteoporotic subjects.

REFERENCES

1. Jones G, Nguyen T, Sambrook P et al. Progressive loss of bone in the femoral neck in elderly people: longitudinal findings from the Dubbo osteoporosis epidemiology study. *Br Med J* (1994), **309**: 691–5.
2. Lau WMC, Woo J, Leung PC et al. Low bone mineral density, grip strength and skinfold thickness are important risk factors for hip fracture in Hong Kong Chinese. *Osteoporos Int* (1993), **3**: 66–70.
3. Peel NFA, Barrington NA, Smith TWD et al. Distal forearm fracture as risk factor for vertebral osteoporosis. *Br Med J* (1994), **308**: 1543–4.
4. Burger H, van Daele PLA, Algra D et al. Vertebral deformities as predictors of non-vertebral fractures. *Br Med J* (1994), **309**: 991–2.
5. Kotowicz MA, Melton LJ, Cooper C et al. Risk of hip fracture in women with vertebral fracture. *J Bone Miner Res* (1994), **9**: 599–605.
6. Hans D, Dargent-Molina P, Schott AM et al. Ultrasonographic heel measurements to predict hip fracture in elderly women: the EPIDOS prospective study. *Lancet* (1996), **348**: 511–14.
7. Seaman E, Hosser JL, Bach LA et al. Reduced bone mass in daughters of women with osteoporosis. *N Engl J Med* (1989), **320**: 554–8.
8. Adebajo AD, Cooper C, Grimley Evans J. Fractures of the hip and distal forearm in West Africa and the United Kingdom. *Age Ageing* (1991), **20**: 435–8.
9. O'Neill TW, Felsenberg D, Varlow J, Cooper C, Kanis JA, Silman AJ. The prevalence of vertebral deformity in European men and women: the European Vertebral Osteoporosis Study. *J Bone Miner Res* (1996), **11**: 1010–18.
10. Hernandez-Avila M, Colditz GA, Stampfer MJ et al. Caffeine, moderate alcohol intake and risk of fracture of the hip and forearm in middle aged women. *Am J Clin Nutr* (1991), **54**: 157–63.

11. Nguyen R, Sambrook P, Kelly P et al. Prediction of osteoporotic fractures by postural instability and bone density. *Br Med J* (1993), **307**: 1111–15.

12. Vetter NL, Lewis PA, Ford D. Can health visitors prevent fractures in elderly people? *Br Med J* (1992), **304**: 888–90.

13. Lauritzen JB, Petersen MM, Lund B. Effect of external hip protectors on hip fractures. *Lancet* (1993), **341**: 11–13.

14. Hoyland JA, Freemont AJ, Jayson MIV. Intervertebral foramen venous obstruction. A cause of periradicular fibrosis? *Spine* (1989), **14**: 558–61.

15. Ralston SH, Urquhart GDK, Brzesky M et al. Prevalence of vertebral compression fractures due to osteoporosis in ankylosing spondylitis. *Br Med J* (1990), **300**: 565–6.

16. Taggart HM, Tweedie DR. Spinal cord compression: remember osteoporosis. *Br Med J* (1987), **296**: 1148–9.

17. Todd CJ, Freeman CJ, Camilleri-Ferrante C et al. Differences in mortality after fracture of hip: the East Anglian audit. *Br Med J* (1995), **310**: 904–8.

18. Sinclair S, James S, Singer M. Intraoperative volume optimisation and length of hospital stay after repair of proximal femoral fractures: a controlled trial. *Brit Med J* (1997) **315**: 909–12.

7 The prevention of osteoporosis and fracture

INTRODUCTION

Some degree of loss of bone is inevitable with advancing age. It is part of the human condition irrespective of sex, race, climate or diet. Bone loss, however, leads to microarchitectural deterioration and structural failure with an increased risk of fracture. The manifestation of that risk is usually dependent on some relatively trivial trauma. Therefore, what needs to be prevented are bone loss, especially if it is precocious or excessive, and falls in later life.

The prevention of osteoporosis could be defined as the achievement and maintenance of a sufficient supply of bone, the strength of which is appropriate to the stresses to which it may normally be subjected at any age. Bone strength in later life is determined by the peak bone mass attained at skeletal maturity and the subsequent rate of loss (see Chapter 2). Fracture is determined by both bone strength and the force of any trauma, usually a fall. Its prevention also requires prevention of falls.

The *primary prevention* of osteoporosis can thus be divided into the four phases of life which correspond to the stages of net bone gain and loss: fetal development; childhood growth; young adult life; and the fourth stage of net bone loss in older people. A fifth preventative category is the recognition and alleviation of other diseases or deprivations which cause secondary osteoporosis (see Chapter 4). *Secondary prevention* of osteoporosis comprises measures to prevent further deterioration in those who have been identified as osteoporotic by bone densitometry or suspected by the presence of a predisposing condition, by osteopenia on a plain X-ray or by having previously sustained a low trauma fracture at an early age, especially a Colles' fracture, which could have been osteoporosis-related. *Tertiary prevention* is for those who have already sustained a fracture of a vertebral body or of a long bone after minor trauma, i.e., those who have a definite clinical manifestation of the disease (Figure 7.1). Tertiary prevention is the same as treatment of established osteoporosis and is dealt with in Chapters 8 and 9.

Intervention at all stages is worthwhile to reduce the risk of fracture and improve the quality of life.

Public health measures

'Prevention implies prediction' and, while primary osteoporosis can be predicted on the basis of past experience in a statistical proportion of a defined population, it cannot be predicted with certainty for the individual. There are two ways in which public health measures might help prevent osteoporosis.

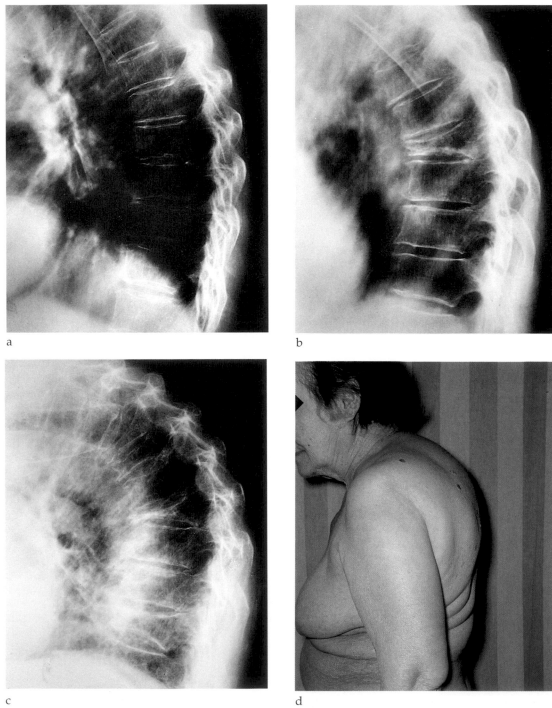

a

b

c

d

Figure 7.1   (a–c) Progressive wedging and collapse of thoracic vertebrae in a postmenopausal woman from the age of 68 over a period of four years. This has led to marked loss of height and kyphosis, and (d) the development of abdominal creases associated with the impaction of the lower ribs on the pelvic brim. Risk factors were menopause at the age of 36 and smoking.

The first is to treat all for the benefit of the few. This requires that the treatment does no harm and is generally acceptable. The second is to screen the population, or a subpopulation such as children or postmenopausal women, in order to identifying those individuals most at risk. For those most at risk, somewhat more in the way of adverse effects of treatment may be acceptable, balancing the benefits against the inconveniences and risks of intervention.

Lifestyle measures

Lifestyle measures that are concerned with building and maintaining a strong skeleton include diet, exercise, alcohol and smoking.

Diet

General nutrition

Undernutrition has many causes such as poverty, famine, ignorance, anorexia and depression. Children in tropical countries[1] and the elderly in westernized societies are most affected.

When total nutrition is deficient the bones suffer along with other tissues. There are multiple depletions and no single nutrient will fully restore bone health. Most at risk of undernutrition in western societies are the frail elderly living alone or in institutions. Poor nutrition

plays a role in their susceptibility to hip fracture and the complications of hip fracture in a number of ways. The effect of lack of calcium and vitamin D on bone mass and fracture is only one of them. Protein–calorie malnutrition leads to weak muscles and poor co-ordination, to loss of soft tissue padding over the hips and is usually associated with markedly lower circulating vitamin D levels, sometimes amounting to osteomalacia on top of pre-existing osteopenia.[2] Lower levels of vitamin C were found in hip fracture patients who developed pressure sores compared with those who did not.[3]

Calcium intake

Calcium intake is often inadequate in western diets and this adversely affects both bone growth and subsequent loss. The recommended daily allowances (RDA) published by the National Osteoporosis Society, UK (which are similar to those in the USA) are shown in Table 7.1. In the UK, the Committee on the Medical Aspects of Food Policy[4] (COMA), recognizing the many factors which affect calcium retention, has abandoned the concept of RDA in favour of dietary reference values

Table 7.1   Recommended daily allowances (RDA) for calcium (National Osteoporosis Society, UK) and reference nutrient intakes (RNI) (COMA)

	Calcium (mg/day)	
	RDA	*RNI*
Young children (1–12 years)	800	350–800
Teenagers (13–19 years)	1200	800
Women aged 20–40 years	1000	700
Men aged 20–60 years	1000	700
Pregnant women	1200	700
Lactating women	1200	1250
Pregnant and nursing teenagers	1500	1250
Women over 40 years (i.e., before, during and after the menopause) without HRT	1200	700
Women over 40 years with HRT	1000	700
Men and women over 60 years	1200	700

and expresses these as Estimated Average Requirements (EAR), Lower Reference Nutrient Intake (LRNI) and Reference Nutrient Intake (RNI). The LRNI is defined as insufficient for all but those with very low needs. The RNI is defined as enough, or more than enough, for 95% of people (Table 7.1).

Concern about weight, lipids and cardiovascular disease has led to caution about dairy intake of milk and milk-derived foods, yet these are the most abundant source of dietary calcium. Low fat or fat-free products contain more calcium per gram as the fat has been removed. Public education is needed to give a single simple message that a daily pint of low fat milk is good for the skeleton and not harmful for the heart. In the past British school children were supplied with free milk at school. There is little doubt that this ensured that many children benefited both from the extra protein nutrition and the calcium content in the years of relative deprivation after the Second World War (see Chapter 2, page 47).

Fortification of bread flour with added calcium is another easy, cheap and harmless way of increasing calcium intake and, even if many bread eaters do not need the supplement, few object to it. Wholemeal bread contains about 84 mg of calcium per 100 g of bread but about half of this is in the bran and wheat germ, which are removed when wheat is milled to provide refined white flour. In the UK, by law, the millers must add calcium carbonate to white flour to bring the total calcium content back to the same level as in wholemeal flour. In doing so the State ensures that poorer people, for whom white bread may be a large part of the diet, receive a calcium supplement irrespective of the rest of their diets (see pages 47 and 214). Since calcium-binding phytates are largely removed in white flour, the calcium in white bread is more bio-available than that in wholemeal flour.

Mineral balance

'Salt is a more important determinant of urinary calcium excretion than calcium intake within the usual ranges of salt and calcium intake' according to a review in *The Lancet*,[5] and calcium will be lost from the bones on a high salt, low potassium diet unless a supplement is taken. Alternatively, calcium-sparing potassium supplements are used, such as potassium-rich table salt substitutes or by eating more fruit and vegetables.[6,7]

Drinking water

A public health measure which can have far-reaching effects, without invoking disapproval from any sections of the public, is ensuring adequate 'hardness', i.e., calcium content, in the drinking water. Burton-on-Trent became the brewing capital of the UK not because of the purity of its water supply (in the sense that distilled water is pure) but because the water contained a favourable combination of dissolved minerals, including calcium. However, other water supplies, particularly those which collect rain falling on non-limestone hills or peaty moorlands may contain very little calcium. The importance that such differences in calcium intake can make was emphasized in the well-known study from the former Yugoslavia.[8]

Other epidemiological studies have produced evidence of significant differences in fracture rates related to daily calcium intake. A potential threat to potable water supplies as a source of calcium and hence to primary prevention of osteoporosis is posed by the growing popularity of bottled spring and spa waters. While many of these have an adequate calcium content of around 100 mg per litre, some are almost calcium-free. In Britain, manufacturers of bottled spring waters are not obliged to print the analysis of the contents on the label.

In other parts of the UK tap water is of doubtful safety. In eastern counties of England, where the water supply depends on underground aquifers fed by run-offs from the cultivated farmlands on to which large amounts of nitrogen fertilizers are regularly scattered, the nitrate content of the water may rise to as high as 100 mg per litre (judged against a naturally occurring nitrate content of about 3 mg per litre). In babies, artificial feeds made up with such water might cause methaemoglobinaemia. There have, however, been no reports of nitrate poisoning in adults. Nevertheless, once people cease to trust their water supply for drinking purposes the consumption of bottled table waters will continue to rise. It will be important to choose those with an adequate calcium content.

Caffeine

A number of studies have found little or no effect of caffeine on bone mineral density, partly because a high caffeine intake is often confounded by low calcium intake, low body weight and smoking. However, a positive association with hip fracture has been reported in two studies.[9,10]

Vitamin D

The role of vitamin D in the prevention of osteoporosis and fracture depends on the dose and on the vitamin D status of the subject. Many elderly, in particular those who are housebound, are vitamin D-deficient and maintaining adequate levels appears to prevent fractures. This is discussed in relation to treatment in Chapter 9.

Fluoride

Of concern to osteoporosis prevention but more controversial is fluoridation of water supplies. The physiological range of fluoride in potable water is narrow, 0.5–1.4 mg per litre, but because the long-term effects of under- or over-ingestion of fluoride may take 20 or more years or more to become evident, there is room for much staunchly held conviction and public controversy regarding the wisdom of adding fluoride to a depleted water supply. Simonen and Laitinen[11] compared the incidence of osteoporosis and hip fracture in two towns in Finland. In Kuopio the water supply had been fluoridated since 1959 to bring the fluoride content up to 1 mg per litre. In Jyvaskyla the fluoride content was low (0–0.1 mg per litre). The demography of the two towns and the composition of the water supplies with respect to other elements were comparable. The incidence of fracture of the femoral neck was significantly higher in Jyvaskyla.

In contrast, ecological reviews of fracture incidence in areas of differing water supply fluoride levels have suggested that there is a possible moderate increase in the risk of fractures at higher levels.[12] There is no increase of fracture risk for fluoride content of 1 mg/litre. These findings are consistent with the increased strength and density and resistance to caries attack of teeth in children in areas where fluoride-depleted water supplies have been fluoridated to a level of about 1 mg/litre.

Other trace elements in water supplies have not been shown to affect the risk of osteoporosis and fracture except in the case of water used in renal dialysis machines where excess aluminium can lead to fractures.

Exercise

Physical loading of bone is essential to the normal growth and development of the skeleton, and bone responds rapidly to any loss of use, especially loss of physical loading. A dramatic example is the loss of bone mass due to weightlessness in space without appropriate exercises. In the elderly, exercise has little effect on bone density but does increase fitness and balance and decreases the risk of falling.[13] In young and middle-aged people, increasing weight-bearing exercise consistently increases bone mass as long as exercise is maintained.

Again, public health education is needed to get this message across and time and facilities made available in the home, neighbourhood and workplace.

Sport

Governmental authorities can intervene in the primary prevention of osteoporosis by supporting and encouraging sports and providing suitable facilities. Now that the great majority of people in affluent societies live in towns, sport becomes increasingly important. Ministries of sport are set up and prowess in sports by individuals or teams representing their towns or countries is of political significance, yet provision of sports facilities in schools and the employment of instructors may have a low priority when money is tight. It is in schools where the lifelong enjoyment of physical exercise can be taught. Sports facilities may be provided for adults, but if regarded as irrelevant or too expensive to be made use of by the same children when grown up, those facilities will be underused. Persuading people to accept the public health measures offered depends on the effectiveness of health education.

Smoking

Cigarette smoking, which includes 'passive smoking', adversely affects bone density. In a study of twins discordant for smoking, for every 10-pack years of smoking the bone mineral content was reduced by 2% in the lumbar spine, 0.9% in the femoral neck and 1.4% in the femoral shaft. The differences were greatest in the most discordant pairs.[14,15]

Smoking has been associated with an increased risk of hip and vertebral fractures, although the data are less clear because it is difficult to separate the effect of smoking from those of low body weight, earlier menopause and generally poorer health.

Alcohol consumption

A low or moderate alcohol consumption has no effect on bone density and risk of fracture, and may be protective,[16] possibly by raising blood oestrogen levels in women. Chronic alcohol abuse is associated with reduced axial and appendicular bone density, a higher prevalence of fractures and is a common association of osteoporosis in males.

Falls and fall-prevention

Most osteoporosis-related fractures, especially those of the wrist, elbow, shoulder and hip follow falls. Falls are a leading cause of accidental death in men and women over the age of 75 years. One in every three of the population aged 65 years or more will experience a fall at least once a year. One in every two over the age of 85 years living at home will fall at least once a year, more if living in an institution. Between 5% and 10% of falls result in injury, the commonest of which is a fracture. Forty per cent of deaths from injury follow a fracture. There have been numerous studies of risk factors for falls and of interventions which can reduce the risk of falls, but surprisingly, because it is counter-intuitive, there is little evidence that removing hazards for falls reduces the incidence of hip fractures. This is discussed later in this chapter in relation to osteoporosis in elderly people.

THE PHASES OF NET BONE GAIN AND LOSS

First phase—conception to birth

The first phase in building up a good bone supply begins in embryonic life. In terms of values per kilogram of fat-free tissue, a 13-

week fetus contains 2.1 g/kg of calcium. This rises to 9.6 g/kg at birth, increasing still further to 22.5 g/kg in adult life. Over the same span the potassium content of human tissue rises only from 38 mmol at 13 weeks, 53 mmol/kg at birth to 69 mmol/kg in an adult.[17] Undernourished mothers will produce babies with weak under-mineralized bones unless their diets are supplemented with calcium. Within wide limits, maternal vitamin D blood levels have little effect on fetal mineralization, but maternal calcium intake is important. Whether such deprived embryos will 'catch up' later if properly fed in infancy and childhood is not known. Some evidence comes from monozygotic twins born dissimilar as a result of the placental steal syndrome in which an abnormality of the placental circulation gives one embryo the majority of the placental blood supply and the other is depleted. Some studies indicate that the deprived twin may never fully make up the difference in later life.

Second phase—birth to the final fusion of the epiphyses in late adolescence

The effects of diet and exercise are predominant in this stage. Prescribing physical exercise is hardly necessary for most young children who are otherwise healthy, but diet is another matter. Calcium, vitamin D and first-class protein are required, although deficiencies of other nutrients, for example of ascorbic acid, can also lead to deficient bone formation. The calcium requirements of the nursing infant are provided by the mother's milk and those of the toddler by food, mainly cow's milk and cow's milk-derived dairy products.

Milk

Public health measures aimed at increasing cow's milk consumption have been followed by startling rises in the growth rate and final stature of children, although other factors may have contributed. Examples include the pre- and post-war provision of free or cheap milk to school children in the UK and the campaign in the early days of the Russian Revolution to increase milk consumption by promoting the widespread consumption of icecream. Remembered milk consumption up to age of 24 correlated with maturity bone density at all measured sites was noted in a Cambridge, UK study.[18] Milk contains approximately equimolar amounts of sodium, which is calciuric, and other minerals, mainly potassium, which are calcium-retaining. The net effect is to reduce urinary calcium loss.

Digestive abnormalities

Lactase deficiency and cow's milk intolerance are not uncommon congenital or acquired abnormalities of digestion. Acquired lactase deficiency has been estimated to occur in 5–10% of north Europeans and adult citizens of North America of European origin, but the prevalence may be as high as 90% in some tropical populations. While cow's milk allergy (often held to be responsible for eczema) may be treated by substituting goat's milk (which provides a similar amount of calcium; Table 7.2), congenital lactase deficiency demands avoidance of dried and liquid milk. The calcium in allowable foods then stems almost entirely from bread, vegetables and potable water and will be deficient unless supplemented. Minor degrees of lactase deficiency may be unrecognized in children, who nevertheless learn, because of diarrhoea, distension or abdominal pain, to avoid dairy products. McNeish and Sweet[19] pointed out that a proportion of children with coeliac disease due to gluten sensitivity also have lactose intolerance (four out of twenty-four in their series). Iqbal[20] found wide differences between different racial groups in the same city in the prevalence of lactase deficiency by jejunal biopsy

Table 7.2   Composition of cow's, goat's and human milk, and cheeses and yogurt[22]

Milk	(mg/100 g)			Protein (g)	Lactose (g)	Fat (g)
	Ca	Na	K			
Cow's[a]	116	55	139	3.2	4.6	3.7
Goat's	129	34	180	3.6	4.8	4.2
Human	33	17	50	1.03	6.9	4.4
Cheese				*Protein(g)*	*Carbohydrate (g)*	*Fat (g)*
Camembert	382	1150	109	18.7	1.8	22.8
Cheddar	750	700	82	35.0	2.1	32.2
Cottage[b]	90	36	95	17.2	1.8	0.6
Parmesan	1140	760	150	36.0	2.9	26.0
Emmentaler	1180	620	100	27.4	3.4	30.5
				Protein (g)	*Carbohydrate (g)*	*Fat (g)*
Yogurt	150	62	190	4.8	4.5[c]	3.8

[a]Pasteurized whole milk; [b]uncreamed; [c]mainly glucose and galactose.
Cheeses are mainly 'acidic', i.e. calciuric, because of the high protein, high sodium, low potassium content. Milks are 'basic', i.e., calcium-retaining, because of the high potassium content. Yogurt refers to natural yogurt, unsweetened. Some manufactured yogurts are products designed to appeal to children and have from 5% to 15% added sugar by weight.

(3% of whites, 55% of Indians, 82% of Afrocaribbeans). This must be borne in mind by those who advocate a return to free school milk. Lactase deficiency is likely to be important in calcium kinetics if it leads to diarrhoea causing increased faecal calcium loss, or to pain and distension causing avoidance of dairy products. A yeast-derived lactase preparation, Lactaid,[21] is a useful means of increasing milk and calcium intake. Dairy manufacturers can provide very palatable yogurts where the lactose has been split into glucose and galactose.

Bread flour

Studies in Northumbria, UK showed that the sources of calcium in the diets of teenage children were: milk (25%); beverages (water, milky drinks) (12%); puddings (including yogurt and icecream) (10%); bread (9%); and cheese (8%).[23] In the absence of calcium fortification of bread flour, the proportion of children whose diets were totally inadequate as regards calcium would have quadrupled. The mean calcium intake in teenage boys was 786 mg/day, compared with the Reference Nutrient Intake of 1000 mg/day. The figures for teenage girls were 763 mg/day (RNI 800 mg/day). Mean intakes obscure the fact that for many children the intake is considerably below the mean, especially in social classes 3, 4 and 5. The period of ages 11–15 is the time of most rapid accretion of calcium in the growing skeleton and deprivation at this time leads to lifelong effects on bones. Moreover, the calcium intake in the children studied was considerably lower than the amount of daily calcium found by Heaney et al.[24] to be necessary to achieve neutral calcium balance in older women on a reasonably affluent, self-selected diet. Calcium fortification of bread flour, therefore, contributes significantly to the minimizing of osteoporosis risk in elderly people, both at the stage of bone formation and later in life when calcium conservation is less efficient.

School meals

In the UK, schools must assure meals for their students. For those meals cooked at school or bought in from caterers, national guidelines for healthy nutrition have been formulated. School meals, by law, are free or subsidized for children of the poorest families, mainly those in receipt of welfare benefits. Other parents must pay for them. With deregulation, certain unfavourable trends are discernible. The income difference between social classes has widened. Over 20% of children now arrive at schools in the UK not having had breakfast, through poverty, pressure on the time of wage-earning parents or, in girls, through attempts at reducing weight.[25] Some inner-city schools are finding that they have to provide breakfast if the children are to be in a fit state to be taught.[26]

School-provided lunches, although of greater nutritional standard, are being replaced, because they are cheaper, by parent-provided packed lunches consisting mainly of sweetened drinks, potato crisps and chocolate sandwich bars, while those children who are entitled to free meals are being given vouchers which they can exchange for a meal at the school cafeteria or, too often, at the tuck shop for sweets. Children eating packed lunches consume an excessive amount of fat, sugar and salt, and their diets are depleted in fruit and fibre and low in iron and calcium. Bad food habits acquired in school tend to become the norm in adult life and childhood obesity encourages withdrawal from sports and exercise.

Calcium supplements for children

Two exemplary studies have provided strong evidence for the value of calcium supplements in addition to a normal diet in children. The first looked at prepubertal monozygotic twins. The index twins of each pair who were given a 1000 mg calcium supplement increased their bone mass faster than their unsupplemented co-twins. The difference was lost when treatment stopped. This indicated that if the benefit were to be maintained supplementation should continue throughout the growth period.[27] Lloyd et al.[28] reported a randomized double blind placebo-controlled trial of the effect over 18 months of prescribed 550 mg calcium citrate malate supplementation on bone density and bone mass in 94 girls aged 11.9 ± 0.5 years. Basic normal diets averaged 960 mg/day increased by an average of 345 mg when supplemented. Increasing the daily calcium intake from 80% to 110% of the USA recommended daily allowance resulted in significant increases in total body weight and spinal bone density. Increases of 24 g of bone gained per year in the supplemented group translated as an additional 1.3% of skeletal bone mass per year during adolescent growth 'which may provide protection against future osteoporotic fracture'. Note that the calcium intake before supplementation was higher than that recorded in British school children (see also page 47 for the effects of milk supplements).

Potassium and other electrolytes in childhood and adolescence

Electrolyte balance is maintained by varying the cation content of the urine. On a high salt, low potassium diet, more calcium is lost in the urine. Milk, fresh and dried fruits, nuts and vegetables are good sources of potassium, leading to calcium conservation.

Fluoride

Trace amounts of fluoride in the water supply are important in this age group (see page 216).

Exercise in childhood and adolescence

The role of exercise in adolescence is universally recognized. Nevertheless, other pressures, academic or cultural, often discourage girls from taking regular exercise, who in later life will be most at risk. Excess exercise in adolescence can be harmful however if it leads to oligomenorrhoea or amenorrhoea.

Idiopathic juvenile osteoporosis

Idiopathic juvenile osteoporosis is both rare and sporadic. Primary prevention is impossible. Secondary prevention, once the condition has been identified, is a matter of the physician's judgement. Since about half of those affected recover, proof of the effectiveness of any drug is difficult. Secondary juvenile osteoporosis is more common as a complication of childhood debilitating diseases, including juvenile chronic arthritis, coeliac disease, asthma and cystic fibrosis. In many, glucocorticoid therapy will be a contributing factor. Drug treatment depends on keeping the primary disease under control and reducing to a minimum glucocorticoid therapy and, where applicable, changing it to deflazacort. Bisphosphonates and calcitonins have been tried empirically, but there is a theoretical risk that osteoclast suppression by bisphosphonates could lead to a failure of bone remodelling, essential for normal childhood growth.

Third phase—young adult life

Maintaining the strength and bone mass of the skeleton requires regular exercise and enough calcium in the diet, as well as a sufficiency of vitamin D or its equivalent in sunlight to maintain calcium absorption. Smoking and excess alcohol, risk factors for osteoporosis, should be avoided. Young healthy women with a high physical activity, high calcium intake lifestyle, showed a 16.6% increase in bone mass compared with similar women who took little calcium and avoided exercise.[29]

Calcium and young adults

The gradual, and to some extent inevitable, loss of bone mass from the peak (around 35 years) is accompanied by a negative calcium balance. The work of Heaney et al.[24] at Omaha has shown that this negative calcium balance of postmenopausal women can be changed to neutral balance with calcium supplements, and while this does not necessarily mean the increment in retained calcium is equivalent to an increase in bone strength, it is a reasonable assumption that it is so.

Amounts of up to 50 mmol (2 g) per day of elemental calcium have been used successfully. There is little evidence that excess calcium in the diet is ever harmful, except possibly in those with idiopathic hypercalciuria and calcium stone formation.

Calcium is not strongly conserved in the human body after the period of growth. Bone is a reservoir from which is drawn the ionized tissue fluid and blood calcium, the level of which is literally vital and an overall negative balance of calcium ingestion with respect to faecal and urinary losses cannot be compensated for simply by switching off the availability of calcium from the skeletal store. In pregnancy and lactation, the calcium needs of the fetus and infant are drawn from the mother's skeleton, however deficient in calcium her diet may be, so maintenance of a high calcium diet for the pregnant and nursing mother is important in the prevention of osteoporosis in her later life.

Oestrogen

Also important, although less subject to medical control, is the total experience in women of the anabolic hormone activity of oestrogen drive, so that early menarche, late menopause and total fertility and parity all contribute to the maintenance of better bones. Supplementing this with oestrogen in the form of low dose oral contraceptives has been associated with an increase in vertebral bone mass.

Alcohol and smoking

Moderate alcohol consumption (social drinking) is associated with a higher bone density in men and women,[16] but excess is associated with reduced bone density and fracture. Smoking is associated with reduced bone mass and increased risk of fracture.

Protein

Dietary phosphate seems to have little effect on bone mineral content, but there is evidence that a diet rich in first-class protein in excess of the body's needs for tissue repair or growth may contribute to osteoporosis. The sulphur-containing amino acids (methionine, cystine, homocystine, cysteine), if present in excess, are metabolized to sulphate, the excretion of which causes an acid urine compensated by increases in the excretion of calcium. Feeding extra protein to normal subjects induces increased calcium loss in the urine and a negative calcium balance.[30] The extent to which this mechanism contributes to the frequency of osteoporosis in people, particularly in women, used to an affluent diet, has not been fully evaluated. However, on present evidence people should not overindulge in meat or fish after the period of skeletal growth, although no precise limits can as yet be given.

Fourth phase—later adult life

Everyone loses bone mass in later life. Net bone loss in women is commonly thought to begin at or around the menopause, but in fact starts earlier (see page 195). Certain conditions are associated with more rapid bone loss, and these must be recognized and priority given to prevention (see page 195).

Hormone replacement therapy after the menopause

The loss of ovarian hormones leads to an acceleration of the normal rate of bone mineral loss. This can most clearly be seen in women who are castrated because of an ovarian tumour. The exact date of loss of ovarian function is known in such women, bone density measurements can be taken before and after and one can establish the rate of bone loss. Perimenopausal acceleration of bone loss can be prevented by hormone replacement therapy (HRT) (see Chapter 8). HRT should, as noted above, be supplemented by adequate dietary calcium, as ageing is associated both with a reduced dietary intake and a relative malabsorption of consumed calcium. For women who are not offered, or who decide against HRT, the advice must be to take regular exercise, an adequate dietary calcium or supplements. Bisphosphonates and selective oestrogen receptor modulators (SERMs) may be alternatives although there are few data at present concerning their use at this stage of primary prevention.

Women at risk of osteoporosis do not consult doctors to maintain bone density, they seek protection against loss of bone strength. Thus, the only relevant outcome measure in studies of therapy in osteoporosis is reduction in the fracture rate. The work of Riggs et al.[31] suggested that the vertebral fracture rate could be considerably reduced by oestrogens alone but more effect was found if calcium supplements were also given. Vitamin D supplements, however, had no consistent effect. One study[32] found that transdermal oestrogen could prevent further fractures in women who already had marked bone loss. Another study[33] found that the same effect on bone conservation can be achieved with half the dose of oestrogen if calcium is given at the same time. Dietary calcium should therefore be evaluated and, if necessary, brought up to a daily intake of 37.5 mmol (1500 mg) or more (see page 216).

Measuring bone mineral density and prevention

Bone mineral density, measured by DXA scanning, can give valuable information as to the need to intervene to prevent osteoporosis or prevent further deterioration of bone mineral mass. *Low bone density* is defined as a T score of less than –1, i.e., less than one standard deviation below the mean for young adults. *Osteoporosis* is defined as a T score of less than –2.5. *Established osteoporosis* is defined as a T score of less than –2.5 in the presence of an osteoporosis-related fracture. The Z score compares the DXA result for the individual with the reference range derived from appropriate age, sex and race population norms.

Patients in the lower quartile of the reference range for hip bone density have a risk of fracture which is eight times higher than those in the upper quartile. The lower quartile includes patients whose spine or hip bone mineral density is less than about 93% of that expected for their ages, or can be defined as a Z score of –0.67. The strength of recommendation for preventive therapy increases as the bone density is reduced but there is no absolute cut-off for when to recommend intervention. Any decision depends on a discussion between doctor and patient of the risks and benefits of osteoporosis and interventions for its prevention. Prevention should, however, be considered if the Z score is less than –0.67. This might be hormone replacement for a woman, or it might be a bisphosphonate such as etidronate or alendronate for a man or for a woman for whom HRT is unsuitable. The

decision should never be made solely on the results of the scan. While low bone density at various sites[34] is predictive of fracture for groups of women, it cannot identify individuals who will fracture.[35] Equally if not more important is a full history and investigation. Some patients have a strong family history of fractures in later life which is a risk factor independent of bone density. In specialized clinics about one in ten patients referred for osteoporosis have an additional precipitating factor such as heavy smoking, or co-morbidity such as hyperparathyroidism, which will also need treatment.

Quantitative ultrasound promises to be a quick and inexpensive method of bone mass measurement. Both speed of sound (SOS) and broadband ultrasound (BUA) attenuation at the calcaneum have been studied in a group of women over 65[36] and have been shown to predict future hip fracture risk as effectively as does DXA (although the methods do not necessarily identify the same individuals). Comparable data in younger postmenopausal women, when preventive treatment is most effective, or in men, are not available. Quantitative ultrasound cannot yet reliably be used for screening as a guide for predicting who is at risk and should receive prophylactic treatment. Various machines have been developed but as yet there is only a weak correlation between them and with DXA measurements. Ultrasound measurements are not internationally standardized. Improvements and further prospective studies will change this.

Men

Men, having started with a bigger bone supply than women, are less at risk from osteoporosis when elderly. As with women, physical activity, and avoiding excessive dietary salt and protein help to protect their bones. About half of all instances of osteoporosis in men have a discernible cause (see Table 4.1, page 86). Alcohol abuse and glucocorticoid treatments are among the commonest, and both are potentially preventable. Testosterone is under study for secondary prevention, as in prevention of fracture of the other hip in a man who has already suffered one such fracture. Evidence being assembled suggests that the effectiveness of testosterone in older men depends on its conversion to oestradiol in the body. Support for this concept comes from studies of older male trans-sexuals, who take oestrogen to retain their preferred gender and have greater bone mass than their male gender peers.

PREVENTION OF FRACTURES IN THOSE WITH OSTEOPOROSIS

Once it has taken place, osteoporosis can be reversed to only a limited extent. Where osteoporosis itself has not been prevented, the risk of osteoporosis-related fractures is related to risk of falls and, for frail elderly people, several contributory factors for falls exist, both medical and social (see Chapter 2). Some of these risk factors can be modified by and for the elderly osteoporotic patient to influence the likelihood of fractures.

There are four types of medical intervention, exemplified below, which have been shown to reduce the risk of hip fracture and which are supported by randomized controlled studies. Controlled clinical trials, mainly in postmenopausal women with osteoporosis, have shown that bisphosphonates can reduce the risks of loss of bone mass and of fracture.[37] They have been licensed for the secondary prevention of osteoporotic fractures of the axial and appendicular skeleton. It should be noted, however, that data for primary prevention and prevention of fractures in osteoporotic men are scanty (see Chapter 9, page 218). Oestrogen, used transdermally in a controlled study of women who already had one or more vertebral fractures, reduced the relative risk of sustaining a further fracture to

RR = 0.39 in the treated group.[32] Lauritzen et al.[38] used impact absorbing external hip protectors in residents of a nursing home who were aged 69 years or older. After 11 months, there were 8 hip and 15 other fractures in those who wore the protectors, compared with 31 and 27 respectively in nonwearers, a relative risk of hip fracture of 0.44 in those wearing protectors. Success depended on compliance with wearing the supporting garment, which has not been so high in other groups. Chapuy and colleagues[39] used a combination of vitamin D_3 and calcium in elderly residents of nursing homes. Treated subjects had fewer hip fractures than controls.

There have been many studies on the physical methods of preventing falls, such as attention to spectacles, footwear and walking aids, as reviewed by Oakley et al.[40] These measures, and attention to home hazards such as poor lighting, trailing electricity flexes and unnoticed floor-level changes can be effective in preventing falls, but have not been shown to prevent hip fracture in individuals living in their own homes.[41]

THE ROLE OF OSTEOPOROSIS SELF-HELP SOCIETIES IN PREVENTION

The increasing threat of osteoporosis, particularly to women, has brought together many individuals, lay and medical, in local and national societies, such as the National Osteoporosis Society in the UK, dedicated to overcoming the problem, not only by raising resources for research but also by propagating the knowledge already available.

Such self-help groups recruit support, in the main, from younger perimenopausal women who wish to retain their muscular and bone strength. These women are informed and keen to take an active part in the management of the societies, although they themselves may not have the condition. Older women who already suffer from osteoporosis also belong but, being older, are generally less active in the management of such societies but benefit greatly from the information and support that the societies offer.

Osteoporosis society members, their friends and their doctors lobby governmental organizations to implement primary preventive public health measures and already action is being taken. On one level, sales of a commercial 'over the counter' preparation of calcium carbonate, intended for self-medication as an antacid, have risen sharply as women have started taking it to prevent osteoporosis. More women, with the support of their husbands, are asking for freedom to choose HRT, subject to medical indications. And, importantly, articles on preventing osteoporosis appear in the lay press, mainly in women's interest magazines as well as being frequently featured in the broadcast media. For information on osteoporosis societies see page 228.

PROVISION OF SERVICES: THE HOSPITAL-BASED OSTEOPOROSIS CLINIC

The effective prevention and treatment of osteoporosis require primary and secondary care working closely together to ensure a seamless service to identify those at risk of, or with, osteoporosis and provide them with appropriate advice and treatment. Hospital-based osteoporosis referral centres are evolving in a number of ways and those that are most successful have developed along the following lines.

Objectives

1) To provide an osteoporosis treatment and assessment service based on DXA technology plus clinical expertise.
2) To educate the public about the need to prevent osteoporosis.

3) To provide postgraduate education about osteoporosis for primary care physicians, pre- and postgraduate students and for nurses, physiotherapists, occupational therapists, radiographers and medical social workers.
4) To empower primary care physicians to take over the management of osteoporosis sufferers. (This is where most sufferers will be attending, and there are far too many to be looked after in hospital clinics.)
5) To conduct or take part in research into osteoporosis, including better methods of diagnosis, treatment and delivery of care.
6) To undertake regular audit of the service's work.

The team

The leader of the team will usually be a hospital doctor. Osteoporosis is a multidisciplinary problem and no speciality of medicine has an automatic right or duty to take on this role. The team leader is most frequently a rheumatologist or a geriatrician, but in specialist hospitals it may be a gynaecologist, an orthopaedic surgeon or a metabolic bone disease specialist who is more appropriate. He or she will, with assistants if necessary, run an out-patient clinic and have access to beds for the more severely affected sufferers or for particular forms of investigation.

Associated with the team will be a panel of advisers, which may include a gynaecologist, an endocrinologist, an orthopaedic surgeon, a casualty surgeon, a geriatrician, a neurologist, a rheumatologist and a paediatrician. They will advise on subjects within their specialties and also take part in postgraduate education.

There will need to be one or more trained radiographers or specialist nurses to operate the DXA facility and to report and record the results. Experience has shown that a higher standard of reliability and repeatability is obtained when operating the DXA machine is restricted to those who have been trained to use the same routines. There will be a need for a nurse to look after out-patients and another to set up liaison with other hospital departments, in particular casualty and orthopaedics. Fracture clinics are a source of peri- and postmenopausal women who have a low bone density and who should be (but currently seldom are) counselled about oestrogen replacement or other therapy and lifestyle changes.[42] An important member of the team is the nurse or volunteer who acts as secretary of the local osteoporosis support group, and who will organize local and public meetings, home visits, a telephone help line, and deal with the media on their behalves and, where facilities are needed but are unfunded, to undertake fund-raising.

In smaller clinics, one person may assume several roles. In larger centres, several may be required to do one job.

PRACTICAL POINTS

- Adequate maternal calcium intake is vital to fetal bone development, and to protect the mother's skeleton. Vitamin D is less important.

- From birth to late adolescence, sufficient dietary calcium, vitamin D, fruit and vegetables and first-class protein, plus plenty of exercise, are necessary for healthy bone formation.

- The same requirements (but without so much protein) continue to apply until middle age. Using potassium-rich table and culinary salt is a convenient way to help preserve a more favourable calcium balance.

- Net bone loss is accelerated at the menopause in women. Preventive treatment in women can involve hormone replacement therapy and calcium supplementation.

- Public health measures include the encouragement of exercise and sport and the provision of facilities. Measures aimed at increasing dietary calcium intake include adding calcium to white bread flour and drinking water.

- In elderly, mainly institutionalized, people, the use of external hip protectors and taking vitamin D plus calcium supplements will reduce the risk of hip fractures.

- The bisphosphonates etidronate and alendronate have been licensed for the prevention of osteoporosis-related fractures of the axial and appendicular skeleton.

- Self-help societies have an important role to play both as fund-raisers and educators. Hospital-based osteoporosis centres can help with this. National osteoporosis societies have been formed in most western countries.

REFERENCES

1. Branca F, Robins SP, Ferro-Luzzi A et al. Bone turnover in malnourished children. *Lancet* (1992), **340**: 1493–6.
2. Heaney RF. Hip fracture: a nutritional perspective. *Proc Soc Exp Biol Med* (1992), **200**: 153–6.
3. Goode HF, Burns E, Walker BE. Vitamin C depletion and pressure sores in elderly patients with femoral neck fractures. *Br Med J* (1992), **305**: 925–7.
4. Report of the Panel on Dietary Reference Values of the Committee on the Medical Aspects of Food Policy. Dietary reference values for food energy and nutrients for the UK. *Report on Health and Social Subjects No. 4.* HMSO: London (1991).
5. Antonios TFT, MacGregor GA. Salt—more adverse effects. *Lancet* (1996), **348**: 250–1.
6. Sebastian A, Harris JT, Ottaway JH et al. Improved mineral balance and skeletal metabolism in postmenopausal women treated with potassium bicarbonate. *N Engl J Med* (1994), **330**: 1776–81.
7. McParland BE, Goulding A, Campbell AJ. Dietary salt affects biochemical markers of resorption and formation of bone in elderly women. *Br Med J* (1989), **299**: 834–5.
8. Matkovic V, Kostial K, Simonovic I et al. Bone status and fracture rates in two regions of Yugoslavia. *Am J Clin Nutr* (1979), **32**: 540–9.
9. Keil DP, Felson DT, Hannan MT, Anderson JJ, Wilson PWF. Caffeine and the risk of hip fracture: the Framingham study. *Am J Epidemiol* (1990), **132**: 675–84.
10. Hernandez-Avila M, Colditz GA, Stampfer MJ, Rosner B, Speizer FE, Willet WC. Caffeine, moderate alcohol intake and risk of fractures of the hip and forearm in middle-aged women. *Am J Clin Nutr* (1991), **54**: 157–63.
11. Simonen O, Laitinen O. Does fluoridation of drinking water prevent bone fragility in osteoporosis? *Lancet* (1985), **ii**: 432–3.
12. Gordon SL, Corbin SB. Summary of workshop on drinking water fluoride influence on hip fracture and bone health. *Osteoporos Int* (1992), **2**: 109–17.
13. McMurdo MET, Mole PA, Paterson CA. Controlled trial of weight-bearing exercise in older women in relation to bone density and falls. *Br Med J* (1997), **314**: 569–70.
14. Hopper JL, Seeman E. The bone density in female twins discordant for tobacco use. *N Engl J Med* (1994), **330**: 387–92.
15. Pocock NA, Eisman JA, Kelly PJ, Sambrook PN, Yeates MG. Effects of tobacco use on axial and appendicular bone mineral density. *Bone* (1989), **10**: 329–31.
16. Holbrook TL, Barrett-Connor E. A prospective study of alcohol consumption and bone mineral density. *Br Med J* (1993), **306**: 1506–9.
17. Lentner C ed. The composition of the body. In: *Geigy Scientific Tables*, 8th Edition. CIBA-GEIGY: Basle (1981), **1**: 219.
18. Murphy S, Khaw K-T, May H et al. Milk consumption and bone mineral density in middle aged and elderly women. *Br Med J* (1994), **308**: 939–41.
19. McNeish AS, Sweet EM. Lactose intolerance in childhood coeliac disease. *Arch Dis Child* (1968), **43**: 433–7.
20. Iqbal TH, Wood GM, Lewis KO et al. Prevalence of primary lactase deficiency in adult residents of west Birmingham. *Br Med J* (1993), **306**: 1303–4.
21. Anon. Lactose intolerance [Editorial]. *Lancet* (1991), **338**: 633–4.
22. Lentner C ed. Composition of foods. In: *Geigy Scientific Tables*, 8th Edition. CIBA-GEIGY: Basle (1981), **1**: 255.
23. Moynihan P et al. Dietary sources of calcium and the contribution of flour fortification to total calcium intake in the diet of Northumbrian adolescents. *Br J Nutr* (1996), **75**: 495–505.
24. Heaney RP, Recker RR, Saville PD. Menopausal changes in calcium balance performance. *J Lab Clin Med* (1978), **92**: 953–62.
25. National Dairy Council. Teenage eating habits: a summary of a survey carried out in conjunction with Youth Express Magazine. London: National Dairies Council, London 24 (1995).
26. Simeon DT, Grantham-McGregor S. Effects of missing breakfast on the cognitive functions of school children of differing nutritional status. *Am J Clin Nutr* (1989), **49**: 646–53.
27. Johnson CO, Miller JZ, Slemenda CW et al. Calcium supplementation and increases in bone mineral density in children. *N Engl J Med* (1992), **327**: 82–7.
28. Lloyd T, Andon MB, Rollings N et al. Calcium supplementation and bone mineral density in adolescent girls. *JAMA* (1993), **27**: 841–4.

29. Kanders B, Lindsay R, Dempster D et al. Determinants of bone mass in young healthy women. In: Christiansen C et al. eds. *Osteoporosis I, Proceedings of the Copenhagen International Symposium*, Glostrop Hospital, Copenhagen (1985), p. 337–40.

30. Parfitt AM. Dietary risk factors for age-related bone loss and fractures. *Lancet* (1983), **ii**: 1181–5.

31. Riggs L, Seeman E, Hodgson SF et al. Effect of fluoride/calcium regimen on vertebral fracture occurrence in postmenopausal osteoporosis. *N Engl J Med* (1982), **306**: 446–50.

32. Lufkin EG, Wahner HW, O'Fallon WM et al. Treatment of postmenopausal osteoporosis with transdermal estrogen. *Ann Intern Med* (1992), **117**: 1–9.

33. Ettinger B, Genant HK, Cann CE. Postmenopausal bone loss is prevented by treatment with low-dosage estrogen with calcium. *Ann Intern Med* (1987), **106**: 40–5.

34. Cummings SR, Black DM, Nevitt MC et al. Bone density at various sites for prediction of hip fractures. *Lancet* (1993), **341**: 72–5.

35. Marshall D, Johnell O, Wedel H. Meta-analysis of how well measures of bone mineral density predict occurrence of osteoporotic fractures. *Br Med J* (1996), **312**: 1254–9.

36 Hans D, Dargent-Molina P, Schott AM et al. Ultrasonographic heel measurements predict hip fractures in elderly women: the EPIDOS prospective study. *Lancet* (1996), **348**: 511–14.

37. Liberman UA, Weiss SR, Bröll H et al. Effect of oral alendronate on bone mineral density and the incidence of fractures in postmenopausal osteoporosis. *N Engl J Med* (1995), **333**: 1437–43.

38 Lauritzen JH, Petersen MM, Lund B. Effect of external hip protectors on hip fractures. *Lancet* (1993), **341**: 11–13.

39. Chapuy MC, Arlot ME, Duboeuf F et al. Vitamin D$_3$ and calcium to prevent hip fractures in elderly women. *N Engl J Med* (1992), **327**: 1637–42.

40. Oakley A et al. Preventing falls and subsequent injury in older people. *Effective Health Care* (1996), **2**(4): 1–16.

41. Vetter NJ, Lewis PA, Ford D. Can health visitors prevent hip fractures in elderly people? *Br Med J* (1992), **304**: 888–90.

42. Gundle R, Simpson AH. Should women attending fracture clinics be counselled about osteoporosis? *Injury* (1993), **24**: 441–2.

8 The menopause and hormone replacement therapy

INTRODUCTION

In women, the menopause, whether natural or artificially induced, is the strongest determinant of loss of bone mass and risk of fracture (see page 49). Hormone replacement therapy (HRT) is the first treatment that controlled trials had shown unequivocally both to prevent postmenopausal bone loss and to reduce the risk of fracture. In the past some professionals have been hesitant to advise HRT, but the picture is changing. Isaacs et al.[1] found that 55.2% of women general practitioners who were postmenopausal had ever used HRT and most were still taking it at the time of their survey. Nevertheless, the menopause is still poorly understood by some of those who treat osteoporosis, although HRT is safe and has other important beneficial effects.

THE MENOPAUSE

Hormonal changes

Menopause (also called the climacteric) means 'the last menstrual period' but the word is also used to describe other symptoms such as hot flushes. In the seventeenth century only 28%

of women lived until the menopause.[2] Now, 95% pass through it and the life expectancy of a woman aged 50 is a further 27 years.

The approaching menopause is signalled by a change in the regularity, frequency, quantity and quality of the menses. This progresses to amenorrhoea, after six months of which only one woman in six will menstruate again. The transition period from a normal menstrual cycle to complete amenorrhoea may last from less than a year to 11 years, with an average of about four years. There is a normal distribution of the age of menopause (see Figure 8.1), with a mean of 50 ± 1.5 years and a range from about 35 to 60 years. The age at the menopause is not influenced by age at menarche.

There is an increase in plasma levels of gonadotrophins with age (see Figure 8.2), with a steep rise at the time of the menopause. Follicle stimulating hormone (FSH) continues to increase for a few years following the menopause and then gradually declines but never falls to premenopausal levels. Luteinizing hormone (LH) levels show less increase so the FSH:LH ratio becomes greater than one.

The failure of the ovaries to respond leads to a fall in circulating oestrogens which further stimulates gonadotrophin secretion. An ovary does not suddenly 'switch off', but becomes smaller, oocytes and follicles become fewer

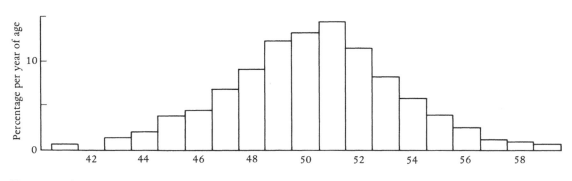

Figure 8.1　Age at menopause.

and replaced by ovarian stroma. Small follicles that do develop soon regress and few viable corpora lutea remain.

As the menopause is approached there is, in comparison to younger women, no change in the levels of oestrogens in the early follicular phase, but in the late follicular phase these are increased, probably because FSH stimulates more follicles into early maturation. Their lower viability results in lower levels of oestrogens in the luteal phase. These large swings in oestrogen levels may account for some of the symptoms of the perimenopause. Oestrogen levels then fall to about 20% of premenopausal values. What causes the ovaries to fail and at what point this causes loss of menstruation remain unsolved questions. The fall in oestrogen levels precedes the menopause but some ovarian activity must remain as levels fall further if oophorectomy is performed less than 4 years after the last menstrual period. Oestrone levels are less affected by oophorectomy.

During the reproductive years, 90% of oestrogens are synthesized in the ovary and oestradiol is the principal circulating form, but after the menopause oestrone levels exceed those of oestradiol (see Figures 8.3 and 8.4). Oestrone can be derived from the androgen, androstenedione. In premenopausal women, androstenedione is derived equally from the

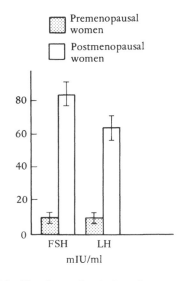

Figure 8.2　The change in pituitary hormone concentrations with the menopause.

ovaries and the adrenal glands. In the postmenopausal woman, the fall in ovarian androstenedione levels means that adrenal androstenedione becomes the main source. The efficiency of conversion of androstenedione increases with age and obesity, as

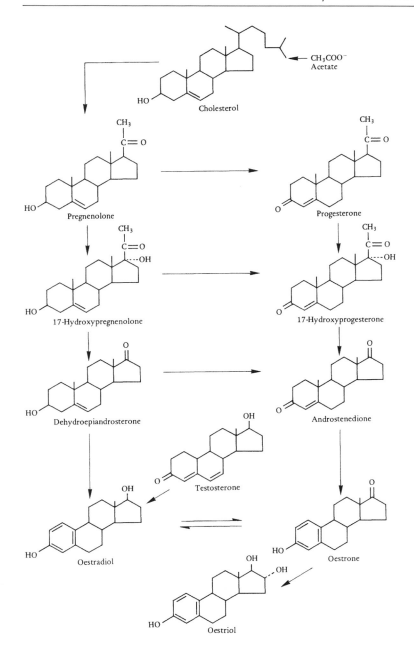

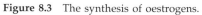

Figure 8.3   The synthesis of oestrogens.

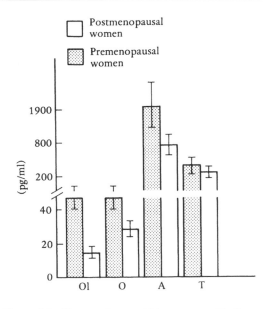

☐ Postmenopausal
women

▨ Premenopausal
women

Figure 8.4 Changes in steroid hormones with the menopause. O1, oestradiol; O, oestrone; A, androstenedione; T, testosterone.

Table 8.1 Menopausal disorders

Autonomic
- Hot flushes
- Sweats
- Palpitations

Psychological
- Mood changes
- Insomnia
- Anxiety
- Depression
- Impaired memory
- Impaired concentration

Reproductive tract
- Atrophic vaginitis
- Dyspareunia
- Reduction of libido

Urinary symptoms
- Urethral syndrome
- Cystitis and pyelitis

Musculoskeletal disease
- Loss of muscle bulk
- Osteoporosis
- Thin skin

Cardiovascular disease
- Coronary heart disease
- Cerebrovascular disease

adipose tissue is the principal site of peripheral conversion. Plasma oestrone levels show a positive correlation with body fat content in oophorectomized women. Postmenopausal women who have little body fat have lower oestrone levels and are more at risk of proximal femoral fractures.

To summarize, at the time of the menopause oestrogen levels at first swing widely then fall to low levels. Postmenopausal oestrogens are largely derived from androstenedione secreted by the adrenal gland and peripherally converted to oestrone. Body fat is the principal site of this conversion.

Clinical aspects of the menopause

There are many clinical consequences of the change in hormonal milieu (see Table 8.1):

- Direct effects on the genito-urinary system;
- Other bodily (somatic) effects of oestrogen withdrawal;
- Vasomotor and psychological symptoms of the perimenopause;
- Effects on the skeleton.

Reproductive system

The vagina and uterus become smaller. The endometrium is smooth but the vaginal epithelium becomes thin and dry with characteristic cytological changes. Vaginal secretion is decreased and its pH increases; the vagina is easily traumatized and subject to infection. Atrophy of the vaginal orifice with loss of secretion is the main cause of dyspareunia. There is some loss of pubic hair, pelvic musculature tone decreases, and there is an increase in stress incontinence and prolapse. There is loss of turgor and of fullness of the breasts.

The epithelium of the urethra and the trigone of the bladder also show some atrophy with oestrogen depletion and cystitis becomes more frequent.

The epithelial changes of the vulva, vagina and urethra and their secretions are reversed by hormone replacement therapy.

Somatic effects

Skin

With ageing and lack of oestrogens there is general thinning of the skin with loss of tensile strength, compressibility and elasticity. There is a decrease in collagen content.

Hair

The postmenopausal increase in circulating androgens is associated with some hirsutism of a male distribution. Some women develop moustache hair.

Heart disease

Premenopausal women have a lower prevalence of atherosclerosis, ischaemic heart disease and acute myocardial infarction than men of the same age. After the menopause the prevalence in women increases to become the same as in men. Of the major risk factors for ischaemic heart disease, hypertension, smoking and raised serum lipids, it is only the latter which alters with the menopause. Postmenopausal women show an increase in total plasma cholesterol, triglycerides and low density lipoproteins.

Chronic diseases

Oestrogen receptors are widespread throughout the body, including the vascular, central and peripheral nervous systems. This may be the physiological basis for reports that hormone replacement therapy is effective in postnatal depression[3] and in women with chronic fatigue syndrome[4] delays postmenopausal loss of muscle strength,[5] reduces the severity or the frequency of relapses in postmenopausal women suffering from multiple sclerosis[6] and Alzheimer's disease,[7] is effective in carpal tunnel syndrome[8] and protects against macular degeneration[9] and tooth loss in the elderly.[10]

Oestrogen accelerates the healing of skin wounds in postmenopausal women, restoring it to the premenopausal rate and opening the possibility that it may help close chronic ulcers.[11]

Perimenopausal symptoms

Untoward symptoms are very common around the time of the menopause. Up to 75% of women suffer hot flushes but only about 20% consult a doctor, of whom over half receive treatment. Perimenopausal symptoms are:

Vasomotor

The 'hot flush' or 'flash' (American) lasts about four minutes and some women experience more than 100 per week. The flush can occur all over the body but usually affects the neck and face. There is a rise in skin temperature, a fall in core temperature and a transient tachycardia. Night sweats may be troublesome. These symptoms are improved with HRT.

Psychological symptoms

In some women the perimenopause is associated with depression, insomnia, irritability, increase in premenstrual mood swings, loss of concentration, loss of libido and reduced sexual activity. Whether all these relate to changes in oestrogen levels or to other factors is unresolved. Sexual problems may reflect vaginal dryness causing dyspareunia with intercourse being painful rather than enjoyable. The loss of libido may also result in sex becoming a 'duty' with feelings of guilt. Controlled studies of HRT have shown a rapid improvement in some of these affective symptoms.[12]

SEX HORMONES AND THE SKELETON

Although the menopause is associated with a variety of symptoms, it is postmenopausal osteoporosis that entails the greatest morbidity and the most serious socioeconomic consequences.

Female sex hormones have an important role in the normal development of the skeleton in women and in the rate of loss of bone mass with ageing (see Chapter 2). Briefly, late menarche and early menopause decrease bone mass; multiparity increases it. Some, but not all, studies have found that bone mass is increased in women who have taken oral contraceptives for at least six months. Bone mass is higher in female athletes who menstruate normally than in their oligomenorrhoeic colleagues.[13]

Albright et al.[14] proposed in 1940 that osteoporosis might follow loss of ovarian function and this has been shown to be true whether the menopause is natural or following castration. The acceleration of loss of bone is most evident after an early surgically-induced menopause.

Bone is lost differentially from cortical and trabecular sites and this determines the likely site of age-related fractures. There is an early increase in the frequency of fractures of the distal radius and then of the vertebral bodies following the menopause and a later increase in the frequency of fractures of the femoral neck (see Figure 2.2). Women are not all equally affected. There are susceptibility differences related to race and genetic factors as well as to lifestyle factors such as smoking and poor general nutrition. However, these characteristics are not specific enough to predict with certainty those who will sustain an osteoporosis-related fracture.

HORMONE REPLACEMENT THERAPY AND THE SKELETON

Historical

An oestrogen was isolated and purified in 1923 and by 1938 ethinyloestradiol and stilboestrol had been synthesized. In the 1950s, long-term hormone replacement was shown to reduce the loss of height in postmenopausal women. In the 1960s, techniques to assess bone mass were introduced. A beneficial effect of HRT on the skeleton was shown in cross-sectional studies using single photon absorptiometry and radiogrammetry. Oestrogen therapy became widely used following this until the mid-1970s when there were reports that it increased the risk of endometrial carcinoma. Later, the addition of progestogen to oestrogen was shown to protect against endometrial carcinoma.

Most studies have been of women in the period shortly following natural or surgically induced menopause, who at entry had no evidence of osteoporosis. The prophylactic effects of HRT rather than its therapeutic effects in established osteoporosis have therefore been the more extensively studied. The effect on bone mass has previously been assessed in the appendicular, predominantly cortical, skeleton, ignoring the effects on the rapid postmenopausal loss of trabecular bone. The various reported studies have used different oestrogens or combinations of oestrogen and progestogen, and are not entirely comparable.

Bone mass

Longitudinal studies of the natural history of bone mass in untreated postmenopausal women are rare. Mole and Paterson, using single photon absorptiometry, followed 67 volunteers for seven years.[15] They found that cross-sectional studies seriously underestimated the loss of bone density in elderly women and that a woman 20 years after the menopause could be losing bone at the same rate as one five years after the menopause.

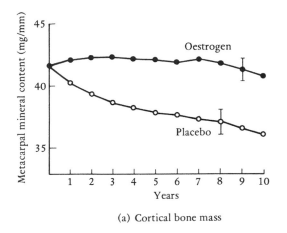

(a) Cortical bone mass

	No. of women with scores of						
	0	1	2	3	4	5	Mean*
Oestrogen	41	13	2	1(1)			0.35
Placebo	14	8	7(1)	8(2)	3(1)	2(1)	1.62

*p < 0.01. Figures in parentheses indicate numbers of patients with vertebrae considered by measurement to have crush fractures.

(b) Spinal scores

Figure 8.5   The effect of HRT on (a) bone mineral content and (b) vertebral fractures in oophorectomized women.

A large group of women who had had bilateral oophorectomy have been followed by the Glasgow Group since the late 1960s.[16,17] Patients were entered into the study up to six years after oophorectomy and were allocated to the synthetic oestrogen mestranol or to a control group. At five years of follow-up there was an increase in the metacarpal bone mass as assessed by photon absorptiometry in women commenced on mestranol. At a mean of nine years after commencement of treatment this protection of bone mass by oestrogen remained, but a small fall in metacarpal mineral content was noted over the final two years in the oestrogen-treated group (see Figure 8.5).

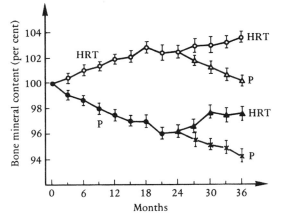

Figure 8.6   Bone mineral content in women treated with placebo (P) or oestrogen/progestogen (HRT) shortly after the menopause in a crossover study.

Christiansen's group[16] have similarly shown an increase in radial bone mass as assessed by photon absorptiometry in women commenced on 17β-oestradiol, oestriol and norethisterone within three years of natural menopause, whereas controls lost bone (see Figure 8.6). After two years, patients on hormone replacement and patients on control therapy were crossed over, enabling these conclusions:

1) With the cessation of HRT, bone loss recurred at the same rate as in those women who had never been treated.
2) HRT was effective in increasing bone mass even if commenced two years after the menopause.
3) All participants were additionally treated with a calcium supplement of 500 mg per day, which did not on its own prevent bone loss.

Other longitudinal studies by Nachtigall,[19] Recker,[20] Weiss[21] and their colleagues have also shown the effectiveness of HRT in preserving bone mass in the appendicular skeleton. In studies that have examined the axial skeleton the results have been similar.[22]

Table 8.2   **Publications showing that oestrogen or oestrogen/progestogen reduce the risk of fracture**

Lead author, year and ref.	Journal	Fracture	Relative risk (RR)	Comments
Hutchinson, 1979[31]	Lancet	hip, wrist	—	E
Lindsay, 1980[17]	Lancet	vertebral	—	E oophorectomy
Weiss, 1980[21]	N Engl J Med	hip, wrist	0.4	E
Paganini-Hill, 1981[32]	Ann Intern Med	hip	0.42	E
Johnson, 1981[33]	Am J Public Health	hip	0.72	E
Kreiger, 1982[34]	Am J Epidemiol	hip	0.5	E
Williams, 1982[35]	Obstet Gynec	hip, wrist	—	E
Ettinger, 1985[36]	Ann Intern Med	all	0.5	E
Kiel, 1987[37]	N Engl J Med	hip	0.35	E
Naessen, 1990[25]	Ann Intern Med	hip	0.79	E, E+P
Almustafa, 1992[38]	Q J Med	vertebral	—	sex hormones
Grady, 1992[39]	Ann Intern Med	hip	0.7	E
Kanis, 1992[40]	Br Med J	hip	0.55	E
Cauley, 1995[41]	Ann Intern Med	hip, wrist, all nonspinal	0.29	

E, oestrogen; P, progestogen.

Established osteoporosis

The effectiveness of HRT in women 10–20 years postmenopause has also been substantiated.[23] HRT has never been shown to increase bone mass by more than about 10%, however. Even if further loss is prevented in a woman whose bone mass is already below the fracture threshold, a theoretical risk of fracture will remain. She will just be prevented from getting worse. However, combining HRT with cyclical etidronate therapy had an additive effect greater than either alone.[24]

Fracture rate

Several case-control studies have shown that long-term oestrogen replacement therapy commenced soon after the menopause is associated with a lower incidence of fractures of the proximal femur or of the distal radius (see Table 8.2).[25,26] A reduction in loss of height and fewer changes in the vertebrae assessed by morphometry have been shown with postoophorectomy hormone replacement[17] (see Figure 8.5). Naessen et al.[25] observed 163 first hip fractures in 23 246 women who had been on HRT during 1977–1980, 41% of them taking oestrogen plus progestogen. This compared favourably with the expected population incidence of first hip fracture of 205.5, a reduction of relative risk to RR = 0.79.[25] Progestogen alone has been shown to prevent bone loss in a short-term study[27] but no effect on fracture rates has been established. The proprietary long-acting progestogen implants used for contraception in young women, Norplant and Depo-Provera, reduce circulating oestrogen levels[28] and in some women have been associated with the development of osteoporosis, which can recover on stopping the drug.[29]

Reduction in the risk of fracture is associated with over five years of HRT and recent users benefit more than do past users.[30] Most studies show that when hormone replacement ceases, bone loss resumes but from a higher level of bone mass than, untreated, it would have been. The effect has been to 'buy time' rather than give lifelong protection.

Table 8.3   HRT: questions to ask

Who?
Why?
When?
How long?
With what?
Who pays?

Summary

HRT stops or considerably reduces the loss of bone mass and protects vertebral bone mass and vertebral height. It is associated with a reduction in fracture rates of the proximal femur, distal radius and the vertebral bodies as long as an effective dose continues for a minimum of five years. Recent users benefit most. The sooner HRT is started after the menopause and the longer it is taken, the greater are the potential benefits.

Postmenopausal osteoporosis must now be regarded as a preventable disease. Since not all postmenopausal women develop osteoporosis one has to identify those most at risk (see Chapter 2), that is, whom to treat (see Table 8.3).

Practical aspects of HRT

Selection of patients

We need better ways of identifying those women whose skeletons are most sensitive to oestrogen withdrawal. The strongest predictor of future risk of fracture is bone density (see page 188). Means to measure this are not always available and in their absence, the identifiable risk factors for low bone density are a reduced lifetime exposure to oestrogen, that is late menarche, early menopause, secondary amenorrhoea, prolonged corticosteroid therapy, a family history of osteoporosis, cigarette smoking, excessive alcohol intake or certain predisposing conditions (see page 57). Oophorectomy before the age of 45 is one of the clearest indications for HRT. Bone markers of rapid turnover and loss may be able to predict who will be at most risk of future fracture, but further data are needed before this is an established method.[42] Baseline measurements of bone density with subsequent follow-up can predict fracture risk but not identify individuals who will have a fracture.[43] Increasing the accuracy of predicting fractures in the individual will need a comprehensive approach which will include clinical and treatment data[44] in addition to measuring bone density and the rate of bone loss.

When to initiate HRT

Neither HRT nor any other treatment can restore more than about 10% of bone mass, once lost. HRT can prevent further loss and is most effective if it is started as soon as possible after the menopause, and may even increase bone mass a little. There is accumulating evidence to recommend its use in women with low bone mass who have already suffered a fracture provided no contraindications are present. Other benefits of HRT, such as increased muscular strength in the prevention of falls, and decreased risk of ischaemic heart disease and stroke need to be taken into account even though the main effect on bone is to prevent further deterioration. Treatment should be commenced as soon as possible postmenopausally, but it is probably worthwhile commencing within 10 years of the menopause. The longer the delay after the menopause, the more other factors must be considered. With increasing age, bone loss is not the major contributor to fractures, it is the tendency to fall, as analysed in Chapter 2. Moreover, a woman of 65 may find it difficult to accept occasional uterine bleeding (with the underlying anxiety of a possible cancer). A major factor in making the decision of their late use used to be whether or not the woman had had a hysterectomy, but with advent of 'no-bleed' continuous-combined forms of HRT this assumes less significance.

Duration of HRT

HRT has been shown to have an effect in reducing the rate of loss of bone after nine to ten years of continuous therapy. However, after six years this effect begins to wane.[17] At present, there are insufficient long-term data to know the optimum or maximum duration of treatment. Some women have continued to receive HRT for over 30 years without apparent disadvantage.

When HRT is stopped, bone loss recurs and when Lindsay et al.[17] studied women who had previous bilateral oophorectomy, they found that this was at a faster rate, which after a further four years negated the beneficial effect of the previous four years of HRT. Christiansen et al.[18] found that a two-year course of HRT in women started shortly after a natural menopause had a beneficial effect over the subsequent 18 months. The Framingham study[37] indicated that past use of oestrogens had some residual protective effect against hip fracture, and a subsequent report showed that benefit to bone mass persisted although it was less marked in those who were aged 75 or more and was greatest in more recent users. In practice, this indicates that the best results in preventing fracture could be obtained by commencing HRT at the menopause and continuing it for life, with a lesser benefit obtained from starting later. Even starting as late as 75 years, HRT could be

expected to confer some benefit but no regime could be guaranteed to abolish the risk of fracture altogether in those who survive to the age of 76 or older. This must be balanced against the increase in risk of breast cancer but decreased risk of cardiovascular disease with more than five years of HRT.[45]

At present, balancing these risks and benefits, the recommendation would be to treat for 10 years or to the age of at least 70 years if the treatment is well tolerated in order effectively to defer postmenopausal bone loss. Benefits still outweigh risks.

Selection of HRT

Many natural, synthetic and semisynthetic oestrogens and progestogens are available (see Table 8.4). Ethinyloestradiol and mestranol have been shown to be effective but natural oestrogens are now preferred. Conjugated equine oestrogens, 17β-oestradiol and oestriol are effective but these have been largely studied in combination with sequential norethisterone or medroxyprogesterone acetate. Transdermal oestrogen preparations and implants are available and have the advantage of avoiding hepatic 'first pass' metabolism.

Combined programmes of oestrogen and progestogen eliminate the risk of endometrial carcinoma (see page 208) and should be used unless the woman has had a hysterectomy. They are either sequential or continuous combinations. Continuous-combined programmes avoid a regular bleed. Hormone replacement therapies that are commercially available and have been found to prevent of bone loss are detailed in Table 8.5. The lowest effective daily dose of oestrogen should be used, such as 0.625 mg of conjugated equine oestrogens, 20 μg of mestranol, 20 μg of ethinyloestradiol or 2 mg of 17β-oestradiol. The dose used should also control symptoms of oestrogen deficiency.

Tibolone is a synthetic steroid which does not provoke uterine bleeding but controls postmenopausal symptoms. It can prevent bone loss.

Table 8.4 Oestrogens and progestogens

Oestrogens

Synthetic	*Natural and semisynthetic*
Ethinyloestradiol	17β-Oestradiol
Mestranol	17β-Oestradiol benzoate
Quinestrol	17β-Oestradiol cyclopentyl-proprionate
Diethylstilboestrol	17β-Oestradiol diproprionate
Chlorotrianisene	17β-Oestradiol valerate
Clomiphene	Oestriol
Dienoestrol	Conjugated equine oestrogens
	Oestrone

Progestogens[a]

Progesterone derivatives	*19-Nortestosterone derivatives and relatives*
Didrogesterone	Ethynodiol diacetate
Acetoxyprogesterone	Gestadene
(17-hydroxyprogesterone	Norethindrone
derivatives)	(norethisterone)
Medroxyprogesterone acetate	Norethindrone acetate
Megestrol acetate	(norethisterone acetate)
	Norethinodrel
	Norgestrel
Natural	Norgestimate
Progesterone	Levonorgesterone

[a]Any substance that can produce secretory changes in an oestrogen-primed endometrium.

Selective estrogen receptor modulators (SERMs), such as raloxifene and draloxifene exert oestrogen-like effects on bone without stimulating the endometrium (see page 227). They are being developed for use in osteoporosis and raloxifene has been approved by the FDA for the prevention of postmenopausal osteoporosis.

Another approach to improve the acceptability of HRT is to use the intrauterine delivery of a progestogen contraceptive device in combination with oestrogen, which results in bleeding in only a minority of cases without evidence of endometrial hyperplasia.[46]

Transdermal adhesive patches with the hormone incorporated in the adhesive enable the dose to be adjusted by altering the size of the patch. Low doses may, however, suppress menopausal symptoms in oophorectomized women without delivering oestrogen blood levels high enough to protect the skeleton.[47]

Mechanisms of action

Oestrogen replacement therapy reduces bone resorption. Oestrogen receptors have been found in bone cells and in blood vessel walls. Both direct and indirect effects on bone cells are likely. Women who are postmenopausal have an increased resorption of bone and are in negative calcium balance. The serum calcium and phosphate levels are mildly elevated as are the fasting urine calcium:creatinine and hydroxyproline:creatinine ratios and total hydroxyproline excretion. These fall with oestrogen therapy and the calcium balance is restored.

Table 8.5   Commercially available combination hormone products

Product	Oestrogen	Dose	No. of days/ month	Progestogen	Dose	No. of days/ month
Monthly preparations:						
Climagest	Oestradiol	1 mg, 2 mg	28	Norethisterone	1 mg	12
Cyclo-Progynova	Oestradiol	1 mg, 2 mg	21	Levonorgestrel	0.25 mg, 0.5 mg	10
Ellese Duet	Oestradiol	1 mg, 2 mg	28	Norethisterone	1 mg	12
Estracombi	Oestradiol patches	50 µg	28	Norethisterone	250 µg	14
Estrapak	Oestradiol patches	50 µg	28	Norethisterone	1 mg tabs	12
Evorel-Pak	Oestradiol patches	50 µg	28	Norethisterone	1 mg tabs	12
Evorel Sequi	Oestradiol patches	50 µg	28	Norethisterone patches	170 µg	14
Femapak	Oestradiol patches	40 µg, 80 µg		Dydrogesterone	10 mg tabs	14
Femoston	Oestradiol	2 mg	28	Dydrogesterone	10 mg	14
Improvera	Estropipate	1.5 mg	28	Medroxyprogesterone	10 mg	12
Menophase	Mestranol (rising dose)	12.5–50 µg	28	Norethisterone	0.75–1.5 g	13
Nuvelle	Oestradiol	2 mg	28	Levonorgestrel	75 µg	12
Nuvelle TS	Oestradiol patches	50–80 µg	28	Levonorgestrel patches	20 µg	14
Prempak-C	Conjugated equine oestrogens	0.625 mg or 1.25 mg	28	Norgestrel	0.15 mg	12
Premique Cycle	Conjugated equine oestrogens	0.625 mg	28	Medroxyprogesterone	10 mg	14
Trisequens (Forte)	Oestradiol	1–2 mg (1–4 mg)		Norethisterone		
	Oestriol	0.5–1 mg (0.5–2 mg)	28		1 mg	10
Three-monthly preparation:						
Tridestra	Oestradiol	2 mg	13 weeks	Medroxyprogesterone	20 mg	14
Continuous-combined therapy:						
Climesse	Oestradiol	2 mg		Norethisterone	0.7 mg	
Evorel Conti	Oestradiol patches	50 µg		Norethisterone patches	170 µg	
Kliofem	Oestradiol	2 mg		Norethisterone	1 mg	
Premique	Conjugated equine oestrogens	0.625 mg		Medroxyprogesterone	5 mg	

One hypothesis is that in postmenopausal women there is either a calcium absorption defect or reduced 1,25-dihydroxy-vitamin D_3 activity. This, and the increases in plasma and urine calcium that have been demonstrated in postmenopausal women, cause a negative calcium balance that has to be restored by sacrificing bone. Another hypothesis is that, in the absence of gonadal hormones, there is an increase in the sensitivity of bone towards the resorptive activity of PTH and 1,25-dihydroxy-vitamin D_3. The data to support these hypotheses are sometimes at odds, mainly because of the technical difficulties in assaying hormones.

Other effects of HRT

Reproductive system

Sequential oestrogen and progestogen programmes cause cyclical bleeding in up to

Table 8.6   Contraindications to HRT

Absolute
- Breast carcinoma
- Endometrial carcinoma (oestrogen-dependent)
- Endometrial hyperplasia
- Pregnancy
- Undiagnosed endometrial bleeding
- Uncontrolled hypertension
- Severe current thromboembolic disease
- Ovarian carcinoma (some types)
- Severe liver disease

As always in medicine, it is a matter of balancing risks against benefits for the patient. HRT may sometimes be considered in the above conditions if the situation is discussed.

Relative contraindications
There is little evidence to support the following as contraindications. But commonsense would suggest extra care and assessment of total risks, including those of *not* giving HRT.

- Myocardial infarction
- Cerebrovascular accident
- Thromboembolic disease
- Familial hyperlipidaemia
- Family history of premenopausal onset of breast cancer
- Liver disease
- Breast dysplasia or family history of breast carcinoma
- Hypertension
- Obesity
- Heavy smoking
- Oestrogen-dependent pelvic disease:
  —Fibroids
  —Endometriosis
- Malignant melanoma
- Acute intermittent porphyria
- Severe migraine
- Severe diabetes
- Renal disease

75% of women. The premenopausal pattern tends to continue, those who premenopausally bled heavily will bleed more than those who premenopausally bled lightly. Bleeding is not always acceptable, particularly if several years after the menopause. One practical compensation is that the date of the next bleed can be accurately predicted. The amount of cyclical bleeding is less when lower, but still effective, doses of oestrogens in combination are used. Continous combined oestrogen and progestogen does not cause regular bleeding but 20% will have breakthrough bleeds during the first six months. Bleeding at other times is an indication for endometrial biopsy. Some older women develop endometrial atrophy on sequential oestrogen and progestogen, and bleeding ceases. Endometrial atrophy is usual with continuous combined therapy.

Hormone replacement may cause periodic breast tenderness, which is worse in older women when starting therapy. Premenstrual tension may return. Some women notice an increase in libido. Patients with cyclical bleeding need to be reassured that they will not be at risk of pregnancy.

Cardiovascular system

There is an increase in plasma levels of clotting factors with oestrogen therapy, particularly with the semisynthetic in comparison with the natural oestrogens. There are also reductions in levels of low density lipoprotein and serum cholesterol and an increase in high density lipoprotein cholesterol. Progestogens counter some of these changes. The risk of coronary artery disease in postmenopausal women is reduced by oestrogen replacement therapy, and a fall in mortality (particularly from myocardial infarction) has been shown[48] with an increased expectation of life from one to three years.[49] Adding a progestogen to oestrogen treatment does not negate the beneficial effects on the cardiovascular system.[50] There is some evidence that there is an increased risk of thromboembolic disease caused by combined HRT[51] (see Table 8.6), suggesting care in starting treatment in those with a known clotting tendency. However, the risk of non-fatal stroke or subarachnoid haemorrhage is unaffected by HRT.[52]

Weight gain

It is not uncommon for women to gain weight shortly after starting HRT but this may in part be caused by temporary fluid retention and in part by feeling fitter and eating more. A 15-year study found that women who used HRT weighed no more than non-users and had the same distribution of body fat.[53]

Breast cancer

Many women perceive breast cancer to be a greater threat than cardiovascular disease or osteoporosis-related fracture, although the evidence does not support this. It is essential that the subject be discussed before starting treatment if long-term compliance is to be satisfactory.

Established breast cancer is often oestrogen-dependent and HRT must not be given unless benefit clearly outweighs risk. Mammography should be advised as part of normal screening before commencing HRT to ensure that no lesion is already present. Several large studies have looked for an increased risk of carcinoma of the breast following HRT, but the results have been conflicting. Breast cancers discovered during HRT have been considered to have a more favourable outlook.[54,55] No survey has shown that treatment for five years or less increases the breast cancer risk but it is generally agreed that after 10 years of HRT use there is an increase in the ascertainment of breast cancer, with a relative risk of about 1.25. On the other hand, a previous analysis of the Nurses' Health study[45] indicated that the breast cancer risk did rise after five years of HRT use and did not support the suggestion from other surveys that these cancers reflect earlier detection of cancers with better prognosis.

Breast cancer surveys have been conducted against the background of wide geographical variations in the standardized mortality ratio for this cancer which is five times greater in England than in Japan and twice as high as in Portugal or Greece. A diet high in animal fat also increases the risk of breast cancer. The US Nurses' Health Study, which followed 95,000 women aged 30–35 for 16 years, analysed the contribution of weight gain plus HRT (34%) compared with HRT alone (5%) to the risk of development of breast cancer in post-menopausal women.[56] At present, there are no controlled prospective and randomly allocated studies which reliably eliminate all environmental and inherited sources of variation between groups. Thus, still unresolved is how much of the apparent increase reflects the more frequent medical supervision of women on long-term HRT, is a statistical increase caused by the drop in other causes of death or is a real effect of the hormones.

A 22-year controlled study of oestrogen and progestogen sequential treatment was reported in 1992.[57] The 168 women who took part in the study were living in an institution for chronic diseases. None of those who had received combined HRT had developed breast cancer but six who had never had HRT had done so. The question of HRT and breast cancer was reviewed by Adami[58] who concluded that 'the epidemiological evidence is reassuring; we can feel a great deal of confidence that the net effect with regard to length and quality of life is beneficial.' An analysis of 90% of the world-wide epidemiological evidence on the relation between the risk of breast cancer and the use of hormone replacement therapy (HRT) concluded that there was a small annual increase (by a factor of 1.023) in the risk of breast cancer but this was equivalent to the increased risk of delaying the menopause. The increase in risk disappeared within 4 years of stopping treatment. 'These findings should be considered in the context of the benefits and other risks associated with the use of HRT.'[59] Benefits outweigh risks on present analysis.

Are women with a family history of breast cancer unsuitable for HRT?

In recent years much progress has been made in the identification of genes which predispose to breast cancer. Nearly all genetically determined breast cancers declare themselves before the menopause. In such a family, a woman who passes through the menopause without developing a cancer will not have inherited the responsible gene. Her chances of developing a cancer postmenopausally are the same as for other women. Similarly, a woman is not more likely, on present evidence, to be predisposed to breast cancer if a female relative developed a breast cancer after the menopause.

Endometrial cancer

Unopposed oestrogen treatment carries a fivefold or greater increase in the risk of endometrial cancer but this is reduced to below the normal expectation if combined oestrogen/progestogen forms of HRT are used. There is no place for continuous unopposed oestrogen therapy in women who still possess their uterus. A progestogen should be combined with an oestrogen for a minimum of 10 days per month, although 12 days is probably better. Using such a combination regime, endometrial biopsies are only required if breakthrough bleeding occurs, that is, bleeding at other than the expected part of the cycle. Breakthrough bleeding may occur in the first three to six months of continuous combined HRT in 20% of cases, but then becomes an infrequent problem. Premenstrual tension may result from the progestogen and trying different preparations may be helpful.

Pelvic endometriosis

Endometriosis after the menopause may be reactivated by HRT and has been associated with ureteric obstruction.[60]

Starting HRT

HRT should not be commenced without a competent examination of the breasts and pelvis, supplemented if need be by a biopsy of the cervix, the endometrium or any suspicious breast lump. Mammography is advisable if available as part of a local screening programme. These precautions are intended to exclude a pre-existing cancer of breast or uterus. Nor should therapy be begun unless the patient has had an interview with adequate time for counselling and full consideration of the facts. In practical terms, there should be, in the health centre or the hospital, a dedicated menopause and osteoporosis clinic or service, with clear lines of responsibility. Whoever is in charge must be able to deal with or refer other women's health problems. Regular follow-up must be provided and records kept. HRT to prevent osteoporosis should not be started if it is unlikely to be continued because of financial considerations, educational attainments, or religious convictions or other factors. Not all women can tolerate HRT. Immediate adverse reactions can persuade them to withdraw from treatment. The most common symptoms are related to fluid retention with temporary weight gain, ankle swelling and feelings of distension. It needs to be explained that these reactions are temporary. If they occur, it is worth trying different preparations. Good counselling by a health professional or contact with someone already taking and tolerating HRT increase compliance.

Who pays?

Currently, in affluent countries, the costs of the prevention and treatment of osteoporosis are borne by the patient privately if she can afford it, by health insurers if they accept the risk, or by the state through its national health service. In all cases the need is to purchase the treatment which is best value for money, keeping in mind the individual's particular requirements. Using published data Francis et al.[61] estimated the annual cost of one averted osteoporotic vertebral fracture to be: for HRT, £130–680 (US$195–1020); for cyclical etidronate, £1880 (US$2820); and for salmon calcitonin, £9075–25 013 (US$13 613–37 520).

As HRT also reduces the risk of heart disease in women it is clearly the preferred option, although one not open to men with osteoporosis. Estimating the costs of averting osteoporosis-related hip fractures illustrates the difficulties of applying health care economics to an area where the benefits may not be seen for a long time and not by all. The savings in terms of avoided hip surgery and improved quality and duration of independent living will be significant, but this is not the whole picture. Prevention of hip fracture at the age of 70 years plus is best accomplished by starting HRT 20 years earlier. However, as only one in five 50-year-old women will be destined to sustain a hip fracture and there are as yet only crude ways of distinguishing who will be most at risk, it would be necessary to treat up to five women for every fracture prevented. Secondly, if a woman lives longer because she no longer dies of the consequences of hip fracture she will survive to succumb to another condition which could be more expensive in terms of medical resources. Thus, net costs may outweigh the savings. Realizing this, econometricians and others are looking at measures of the quality of life and of the 'compression of preterminal morbidity', i.e., the prolongation of healthy, independent life as opposed to mere survival.

PRACTICAL POINTS

- The menopause is associated with an accelerated rate of bone loss and increased risk of fracture. Medically and socioeconomically, postmenopausal osteoporosis is the most serious of the menopausal symptoms.

- Hormone replacement therapy will maintain cortical bone mass after the menopause and remains effective for as long as it is given. In practice, it is best started as soon as possible after the menopause but can be initiated at any time after the menopause providing it is acceptable to the woman. It protects against loss of vertebral trabecular bone mass and vertebral height and is associated with a reduction in the fracture rates of the proximal femur, distal radius and vertebral bodies.

- Risk factors for osteoporosis and fracture are: a low bone density, reduced lifetime exposure to oestrogen, corticosteroid therapy, smoking, excess alcohol, family history of osteoporosis and certain predisposing conditions.

- The risk of endometrial carcinoma is minimized if a progestogen is combined with an oestrogen for at least 10 days per month.

- In considering HRT and its risks, remember the high mortality of unprevented osteoporosis and the benefits with regard to cardiovascular disease and the duration and quality of that life.

REFERENCES

1. Isaacs AJ, Britton AR, McPherson K. Utilisation of hormone replacement therapy by women doctors. *Br Med J* (1995), **311**: 1399–1401.

2. Studd JWW, Chakravarti S, Oram D. Practical problems in the treatment of the climacteric syndrome. *Postgrad Med J* (1976), **52** (suppl 6): 60–4.

3. Gregoire AJP, Kumar R, Everitt B et al. Transdermal oestrogen for treatment of severe postnatal depression. *Lancet* (1996), **347**: 930–3.

4. Studd J, Panay N. Chronic fatigue syndrome. *Lancet* (1996) **348**: 1364.

5. Philips SK, Rook KM, Siddle NC et al. Muscle weakness in women occurs at earlier age than in men but strength is preserved by hormone replacement therapy. *Clin Sci* (1993), **84**: 95–8.

6. Smith R, Studd JWW. A pilot study of the effect upon multiple sclerosis of the menopause, hormone replacement therapy and the menstrual cycle. *J R Soc Med* (1992), **85**: 612–13.

7. Tang M-X, Jacobs D, Stern Y et al. Effect of oestrogen during menopause on risk and age of onset of Alzheimer's disease. *Lancet* (1996), **348**: 429–32.

8. Confino-Cohen R, Lishber M, Savin H et al. Response of carpal tunnel syndrome to hormone replacement therapy. *Br Med J* (1991), **303**: 1514.

9. Eye Disease Case-control Study Group. Risk factors for neovascular age-related macular degeneration. *Arch Ophthalmol* (1992), **110**: 1701–8.

10. Krall EA, Dawson-Hughes B, Hannon MT, Wilson PWF, Kiel DP. Postmenopausal estrogen replacement and tooth retention. *Am J Med* (1997), **102**: 536–42.

11. Ashcroft G. *Nature Med* (1997) **3**: 1209–15.

12. Fedor-Freybergh P. The influence of oestrogens on the well-being and mental performance in climacteric and postmenopausal women. *Acta Obstet Gynecol Scand* (1977), **64**: 1–66.

13. Drinkwater BL, Nilson K, Chesnut CH et al. Bone mineral content of amenorrheic and eumenorrheic athletes. *N Engl J Med* (1984), **311**: 277–81.

14. Albright F, Bloomberg E, Smith PH. *Trans Assoc Am Physicians* (1940), **55**: 298–305.

15. Mole PA, Paterson C. Seven-year longitudinal study of bone density in postmenopausal women. *Bone* (1996) **16**: 679–95.

16. Lindsay R, Hart DM, Aitken JM et al. Long-term prevention of postmenopausal osteoporosis by oestrogen. *Lancet* (1976), **i**: 1038–40.

17. Lindsay R, Hart DM, Forrest C et al. Prevention of spinal osteoporosis in oophorectomised women. *Lancet* (1980), **ii**: 1151–4.

18. Christiansen C, Christensen MS, Transbol I. Bone mass in postmenopausal women after withdrawal of oestrogen/progestogen therapy. *Lancet* (1981), **i**: 459–61.

19. Nachtigall LF, Nachtigall RH, Nachtigall RD et al. Oestrogen replacement therapy: a ten-year prospective study in the relationship to osteoporosis. *Obstet Gynaecol* (1979), **53**: 277–81.

20. Recker RR, Saville PC, Heaney RP. Effect of estrogen and calcium carbonate on bone loss in postmenopausal women. *Ann Intern Med* (1977), **87**: 649–55.

21. Weiss NS, Ure CL, Ballard J. Decreased risk of fracture of the hip and forearm with postmenopausal use of estrogen. *N Engl J Med* (1980), **303**: 1195–9.

22. Genant HK, Cann C, Ettinger B et al. Quantitative computed tomography of vertebral spongiosa: a sensitive method of detecting early bone loss after oophorectomy. *Ann Intern Med* (1982), **97**: 699–705.

23. Quigley MET, Martin PL, Burnier AM et al. Estrogen therapy arrests bone loss in elderly women. *Am J Obstet Gynecol* (1987), **156**: 1516–23.

24. Wimalawansa SJ. Combined therapy with estrogen and etidronate has an additive effect on bone mineral density in the hip and vertebrae: four-year randomised study. *Am J Med* (1995), **99**: 36–42.

25. Naessen T, Persson I, Adami H-O, Bergstrom R et al. Hormone replacement therapy and risk for first fracture. *Ann Intern Med* (1990), **113**: 95–103.

26. Munk-Jensen N, Pors Neilsen S, Obel EB et al. Reversal of postmenopausal bone loss by oestrogen and progestogen: a double blind placebo controlled study. *Br Med J* (1988), **296**: 1150–2.

27. Lindsay R, Hart DM, Purdie D et al. Comparative effects of oestrogen and progestogen on bone loss in postmenopausal women. *Clin Soc Mol Med* (1978), **54**: 193–5.

28. Rowe PM. Investigations into long acting contraceptives. *Lancet* (1995), **346**: 693.

29. Cundy T, Cornish J, Evans MC et al. Recovery of bone density in women who stop using

medroxyprogesterone acetate. *Br Med J* (1994), **308**: 247–8.

30. Felson DT, Zhang Y, Hannan MT et al. The effect of postmenopausal estrogen therapy in elderly women. *N Engl J Med* (1993), **329**: 1141–6.

31. Hutchinson TA, Polansky SM, Feinstein AR. Postmenopausal estrogens protect against fractures of hip and distal radius: a case control study. *Lancet* (1979), **ii**: 705–9.

32. Paganini-Hill A, Ross RK, Gerkins VR et al. Menopausal estrogen therapy and hip fractures. *Ann Intern Med* (1981), **95**: 28–31.

33. Johnson RE, Sprecht EE. The risk of hip fracture in postmenopausal females with and without estrogen drug exposure. *Am J Public Health* (1981), **71**: 138–44.

34. Kreiger N, Kelsey JL, Holford TR et al. An epidemiological study of hip fracture in postmenopausal women. *Am J Epidemiol* (1982), **116**: 141–8.

35. Williams AR, Weiss NS, Ure CL et al. Effect of weight, smoking and estrogen use on the risk of hip and forearm fractures in postmenopausal women. *Obstet Gynecol* (1982), **60**: 695–9.

36. Ettinger B, Genant HK, Cann C. Long term estrogen replacement therapy prevents bone loss and fractures. *Ann Intern Med* (1985), **102**: 319–24.

37. Kiel DP, Felson DT, Anderson JJ et al. Hip fractures and the use of estrogens in postmenopausal women: the Framingham study. *N Engl J Med* (1987), **317**: 1169–74.

38. Almustafa M, Doyle FH, Gutteridge DJ et al. Effects of treatment by calcium and sex hormones on vertebral fracturing in osteoporosis. *Q J Med* (1992), **300**: 283–94.

39. Grady D, Rubin SM, Petitti DB et al. Hormone therapy to prevent disease and prolong life in post menopausal women. *Ann Intern Med* (1992), **117**: 1016–37.

40. Kanis JA, Johnell O, Gullberg B et al. Evidence for efficacy of drugs affecting bone metabolism, in preventing hip fracture. *Br Med J* (1992), **305**: 1105.

41. Cauley JA, Seeley DG, Ensrud K et al. Estrogen replacement therapy and fractures in older women. *Ann Intern Med* (1995), **122**: 9–16.

42. Christiansen C, Riis BJ, Rodbrø P. Prediction of rapid bone loss in osteoporosis. *Lancet* (1987), **i**: 1105.

43. Marshal D, Johnel O, Wedel H. Meta-analysis of how well measures of bone mineral density predict occurrence of osteoporotic fractures. *Br Med J* (1996), **312**: 1254–9.

44. Dargent-Molina P, Favier F, Grandjean H et al. Fall-related factors and the risk of hip fracture: the EPIDOS prospective study. *Lancet* (1996), **348**: 145–8.

45. Colditz GA, Hankinson SE, Hunter DJ et al. The use of estrogens and progestins and the risk of breast cancer in postmenopausal women. *N Engl J Med* (1995), **332**: 1589–93.

46. Anderson K, Mattson LA, Rybo G et al. Intrauterine release of levonorgestrel: a new way of adding progestogen in hormone replacement therapy. *Obstet Gynaecol* (1992), **79**: 963–7.

47. Anderson CHM, Raju SK, Forsling ML et al. Oestrogen replacements after oophorectomy: comparison of patches and implants. *Br Med J* (1992), **305**: 90–1.

48. Bush TL, Cowan LD, Barret-Connor E et al. Estrogen use and all-cause mortality. *JAMA* (1983), **240**: 903–6.

49. Henderson BE, Paganini-Hill A, Ross RK. Decreased mortality in users of estrogen replacement therapy. *Arch Intern Med* (1991), **151**: 75–8.

50. Medical Research Council's General Practice Research Framework. Randomised comparison of oestrogen versus oestrogen plus progestogen hormone replacement therapy in women with hysterectomy. *Br Med J* (1996), **312**: 473–8.

51. Vandenbrouke JP, Helmerhorst FM. Risk of venous thrombosis with hormone replacement therapy [Editorial Commentary]. *Lancet* (1996), **348**: 972.

52. Pedersen AJ, Lidegaard O, Kreiner S et al. Hormone replacement therapy and risk of non-fatal stroke. *Lancet* (1997) **350**: 1277–83.

53. Kritz-Silverstein D, Barrett-Connor E. Long-term postmenopausal hormone use, obesity, and fat distribution in older women. *JAMA* (1996), **275**: 46–9.

54. Harding D, Knox WF, Faragher EB et al. Hormone replacement therapy and tumour grade in breast cancer: a prospective study in a screening unit. *Br Med J* (1996), **312**: 1646–7.

55. Salmon RJ, Remvikos Y, Ansquer Y et al. HRT and breast cancer. *Lancet* (1995), **364**: 1072–3.

56. Zhiping H, Hankinson S, Colditz G et al. Dual effects of weight and weight gain on breast cancer risk. *J Amer Med Assoc* (1997) **278**: 1407–11.

57. Nachtigall MJ, Smilen SW, Nachtigal RD et al. Incidence of breast cancer in a 22-year study of women receiving estrogen-progestin replacement therapy. *Obstet Gynecol* (1992), **80**: 827–30.

58. Adami HO, Persson I. Hormone replacement and cancer. A remaining controversy? [Editorial], *JAMA* (1995), **274**: 178–9.

59. Collaborative Group on Hormonal Factors in Breast Cancer. Breast cancer and hormone replacement therapy: collaborative re-analysis of data from 51 epidemiological studies of 52 705 women with breast cancer and 108 411 women without breast cancer. *Lancet* (1997) **350**: 1047–59.

60. Brough RJ, O'Flynn K. Recurrent pelvic endometriosis and bilateral ureteric obstruction associated with hormone replacement therapy. *Br Med J* (1996), **312**: 1221–2.

61. Francis RM, Anderson FH, Torgerson DJ. A comparison of the effectiveness and cost of treatment for vertebral fractures in women. *Br J Rheumatol* (1995), **34**: 1167–71.

9 Medical treatment other than HRT

INTRODUCTION

This chapter is concerned with the treatment of established osteoporosis, that is, the patient who has a low bone mass or an age-related fracture. The aim is to prevent further fracture, in addition to pain control and maximizing function and independence if a fracture has been sustained. As yet, no treatment can make bones grow in mass and strength safely and continuously while the treatment is being given. Some produce a slight rise in bone mass, but seldom more than 10%. Others stop bone loss or reduce the rate of bone loss. An increase in bone mass does not necessarily result in a reduction in fracture risk. This must be demonstrated separately. It is necessary to look at data on all treatments critically.

Questions that must be asked of any study that purports to show that a drug or procedure benefits osteoporosis are:

- Was it a randomized, controlled study, designed to distinguish the effects of treatment from those of chance variation?
- What subjects were studied and how were they selected?
- If women, how long after the menopause?
- Had they sustained a fracture in the past or not?
- How many patients were studied and for how long?
- What was the power of the study?
- What treatment was given to the controls? Were calcium and vitamin D intake standardized?
- Were the outcome measures based on biochemical or histological evidence of bone formation, on increases in cortical or trabecular bone mass, or on reduction of further fracture incidence?

The randomized, controlled trial with the end-points bone mass or fracture rate, is essential to prove efficacy. Bone mass, however, changes slowly and fractures are unpredictable and uncommon. These are facts of life. Because of these factors, adequate trials of candidate treatments for osteoporosis are difficult to mount. To show that a treatment reduces the risk of future fractures requires long-term studies of large numbers of at-risk individuals. Demonstrating a beneficial effect on bone mass is also not without difficulty. A woman aged 70 years might have as little as 50% of the bone mass she had at 20 years, an average loss of 1% per annum. Yet measurements of bone mass seldom have an error of less than 3%. Even in rapidly deteriorating osteoporosis, serial observations over at least a year in a large group of subjects, some treated, some controls, would be necessary to establish effectiveness. Multicentre trials are usually needed. The number of subjects available and willing to take part in such studies is limited. Commercial bias intrudes, companies preferring to support studies of those products likely to produce the greatest rewards. Competition for resources is such that new treatments have difficulty in recruiting subjects for trials.

Despite these hurdles, considerable progress has been made in clarifying the role of bone-active treatments over the last 10 years.

CALCIUM

The most obvious deficiency of osteoporotic bones is calcium, so it would seem logical to increase dietary calcium intake. If this is done, within a few months neither improvement nor arrest of deterioration is detectable using current measurement techniques. This contrasts with the relative ease with which the effect of hormone replacement therapy (HRT) can be demonstrated in recently castrated women. The rationale for ensuring an adequate dietary supply of calcium has been previously discussed (see page 47). Dietary calcium deficiency, if severe enough, leads to osteoporosis in experimental animals, and in man there is a decreased hip fracture rate associated with a high calcium intake.[1,2] Women on a self-selected diet are often in negative calcium balance and this net daily calcium loss increases after the menopause. In both pre- and postmenopausal women, neutral balance can be achieved by supplementation with calcium to a total daily calcium intake of about 25 mmol (1000 mg) premenopausally or 37.5 mmol (1500 mg) postmenopausally.[3] Increasing calcium intake to the point where there is a net positive balance does not necessarily mean that the retained calcium goes into bones. Logically, it might equally well be lodged in extra-osseous tissues—especially the aorta. Even if the calcium is restored to the bones and this result can be shown by improved bone density, it does not follow that the strength of the skeleton has been restored, although this is a reasonable assumption.

There have been a large number of studies examining the effect of dietary or supplemental calcium on bone mass and fracture risk. The majority of these show a positive effect in postmenopausal women except within the first few years of the menopause[4] when the negative effect of oestrogen withdrawal is so strong. Bone mass is increased[5-7] and this is most marked in those with a low calcium intake.[5] An inverse relationship of dietary calcium with subsequent risk of hip fracture has been demonstrated in men and women.[2] The epidemiologic study of hip fractures in Mediterranean countries found a reduced risk of hip fractures in women who had taken pharmacological amounts of calcium,[8] and a randomized, controlled trial found a reduction of new vertebral fractures with calcium supplementation.[9] Other studies have come to the same conclusion.[10,11]

The conclusion is that it is important to ensure an adequate calcium intake of 1000–1500 mg/day in postmenopausal women, either by diet or supplementation to maintain bone mass and reduce risk of fracture, but supplementation beyond this amount is of uncertain value. Calcium is not the most effective treatment and is mainly used as a co-therapy in those with osteoporosis.

Calcium preparations

If it is not possible to achieve an adequate dietary intake, then there is a wide choice of calcium supplements available either by prescription under the National Health Service in the UK or which can be purchased 'over the counter'. Some of these also contain supplements of vitamin D. 'Over the counter' products may additionally contain other vitamins or minerals.

Sufficient calcium should be taken to supplement the likely dietary intake to provide the recommended daily intake (see Table 7.1). Less will be needed if the ideal of raising the calcium content of the diet can be achieved by increasing the proportion of milk, cheese and vegetables consumed.

There is little evidence of hazardous overdosage from calcium supplementation. The formation of calcium-containing stones in the urinary tract is advised as a contraindication to calcium therapy but there are few data to support this. The precipitation in the urinary tract of calcium-containing concretions is influenced much more by hypercalciuria, hypocitricaciduria, hyperparathyroidism or urinary infection than by dietary calcium.

Increasing calcium intake is far more important than the differences between which formulation is used. Supplements can be given in the form of the bone extract microcrystalline hydroxyapatite, or as various salts such as carbonates, citrates, gluconates, lactates and phosphates. It has been said that the chemical form in which calcium is presented is not important as long as it is nontoxic. All the salts are readily absorbed. The chalk cliffs of Dover might do just as well! Finely powdered precipitated calcium carbonate is the basis of most calcium supplements and also of commonly available antacids. Long-term administration of calcium as the carbonate could in theory lead to alkalosis, but in practice this is not a problem. Calcium lactate gluconate has the advantage that it is soluble in water and makes ionized calcium available quickly. The absorption of calcium citrate is independent of gastric acid secretion and is preferable in patients with achlorhydria. Microcrystalline hydroxyapatite compound consists of the mineral from young beef bone. The microcrystalline structure makes calcium readily available to the intestinal calcium transport mechanisms and it is accompanied by a physiological amount of phosphate. There is no possibility of it causing alkalosis. It contains bone matrix protein residues including bone growth factors and increases bone formation in models of bone healing.

Where subclinical vitamin D deficiency is suspected, such as a disabled elderly person who seldom gets out into the sun, a recommended dose is 400–800 IU of vitamin D daily in addition to calcium. This improves calcium absorption and will do no harm if deficiency is not present. Several preparations of calcium with vitamin D_3 are available.

Dietary calcium (see also Chapter 2, page 47, and Chapter 7, page 179)

The chief sources of dietary calcium are milk, cheese, icecream and yogurt (Tables 1.3 and 7.2). It is more acceptable for overall public health to recommend low fat products. Leafy vegetables and nuts are also good calcium sources, while meat and fish are not. Most bottled spring waters are a good source as they contain about 2.5 mmol (100 mg) of calcium per litre but some are almost calcium-free. In hard water districts drinking water taken directly from the tap is a source of calcium but not after boiling it to make tea or coffee, because of the precipitation of calcium-containing scale in the kettle. Orange juice and other fruit juices generally contain calcium equivalent to potable hard water but the extra sugar may be inadvisable in obese subjects.

Directly or indirectly, milk normally provides 50–80% of the adult European calcium recommended daily allowance (RDA). However, the consumption of milk products is steadily declining (from 4½ to 2½ pints (2.56–1.42 litres) per person per week in the UK since the war, partly because of worries about saturated fats and the risk of heart disease. Skimmed, semi-skimmed and partly skimmed milks fortified with skimmed milk powder are now available. The calcium content of such milks is marginally higher per litre than that of raw milk. Milk contains roughly equimolar amounts of potassium, calcium and sodium. The effect of the potassium is to reduce the urinary loss of calcium.

Processed milk products are an important source of calcium. Cheese is made from milk by coagulating the casein in milk, expressing the whey and adding salt. The calcium remains, bound to the milk proteins and peptides. Cheese is the richest food source of calcium. Most of the potassium content is removed with the whey. The high salt content increases the renal excretion of calcium. The original lactose content of the milk is also removed with the whey. Traditional yogurts have the same mineral balance as milk but the lactose content is reduced by fermentation. Dairy icecream is based on milk, eggs and sugar, and nondairy icecream on skimmed milk powder, sugar and vegetable fat.

The existence of subpopulations which are lactase deficient and the altered proportions of minerals in cheeses mean that milk and milk products cannot be looked upon simplistically as merely dietary forms of calcium supplements.

Calcium and osteoporosis subgroups

Calcium and liver disease-associated osteoporosis

Osteoporosis is common in haemochromatosis, alcoholic liver disease, chronic active hepatitis and is almost inevitable in primary biliary cirrhosis (PBC). Epstein et al.[12] treated 64 postmenopausal women with PBC with monthly injections of 100 000 IU vitamin D to diminish any coincidental osteomalacia and randomly allocated them into three groups. The controls received no calcium supplement and the other groups received either an effervescent calcium lactate gluconate supplement equivalent to 40 mmol of calcium or hydroxyapatite equivalent to 35 mmol of calcium. After a mean of 14 months, cortical bone mass was assessed by the metacarpal index and both calcium supplemented groups fared significantly better than did the controls who lost bone. The calcium lactate gluconate group maintained but the hydroxyapatite group gained bone.

Calcium and glucocorticoid-induced osteoporosis

Calcium supplements have been given to glucocorticoid-treated rheumatoid arthritis patients[13,14] with some advantage over untreated controls, but are normally used as co-therapy with more effective agents.

FLUORIDE

Fluorine is a trace element, minute amounts of which are essential for building caries-resistant teeth. Epidemiological studies have shown increased bone densities in people living in areas with a higher fluoride content in the drinking water when compared with areas served by fluoride-depleted water supplies.[15] Fluorosis, described in 1932,[16] results from much higher levels of fluorine ingestion and is seen as pathologically increased density of bones on X-ray. Dietary intake of fluoride is about 3 mg daily, depending mainly on the fluoride content of drinking water. The optimum level of fluoride in the water supply is 1 mg per litre, with a range from 0.5 mg to 4 mg (0.5 mg to 2 mg in hot climates). Other significant sources are tea-drinking and fluorided dental pastes. Fluoride is well absorbed with over 50% retained in the skeleton. It accumulates in bone mineral and teeth, substituting hydroxyapatite with fluoroapatite, the larger crystal size of which may help resist dental caries and bone resorption. Approximately two years are needed to saturate the skeleton with fluoride. It also stimulates bone formation.

A review of the relationship of drinking water fluoride to hip fractures[17] found that the ability to draw conclusions from then available ecological data was severely limited. Some studies suggested that there were fewer hip fractures in districts with optimum amounts of fluoride in the water supply (compared with districts with depleted water supplies), others did not.

Fluoride was first used to treat osteoporosis in 1961. There have been numerous studies of its action. Many of these have been uncontrolled. Various doses and formulations of fluoride in combinations with calcium, vitamin D or oestrogens have been employed. The total body calcium assessed by neutron activation analysis is unchanged by fluoride given in therapeutic doses. Bone density studies have demonstrated an increase in lumbar bone mineral content but that of cortical bone in the appendicular skeleton showed no change or even a decrease following fluoride therapy. These findings suggest that fluoride therapy redistributes calcium from cortical to trabecular bone. An increased incidence of hip fracture in osteoporotic women treated with fluoride has been observed,[18] which would be in keeping with such a redistribution.

Randomized, controlled trials of patients with established spinal osteoporosis, using as end-points the incidence of further fractures of spinal or appendicular bone, have given conflicting results partly explicable by different dosages.[19,20] Adverse effects are common even if daily doses of 50 mg of sodium fluoride (fluoride ion dosage of 16 mg/day) are not exceeded. Gastro-intestinal upsets, painful transient synovitis and painful areas in the lower legs and feet corresponding to 'hot spots' on technetium bone scanning, attributed to stress fractures, occur. Higher therapeutic doses may increase appendicular fractures.[19] Lower doses are less troublesome but risk being ineffective. The balance of the evidence is that fluoride may reduce the likelihood of further osteoporotic spinal fractures but may increase the risk of limb fractures. Fluoride is now seldom used.

CALCITONIN

Calcitonins in their various forms are strongly conserved in nature. In fish that migrate between salt and fresh water they serve to readjust the internal ionic balance against changes in the salinity of the water passing over the gills. Hence salmon and eels are good sources. All calcitonins have much the same action in man and can be regarded as osteoclast inhibitors, reducing calcium absorption from the bones and reducing raised blood calcium levels in hypercalcaemia. In this their action opposes that of parathyroid hormone (PTH). Human calcitonin is a polypeptide hormone containing 32 amino acids secreted by the parafollicular cells of the thyroid. It inhibits bone resorption both in vivo and in vitro. Immunoassays measure different forms. Basal levels of circulating calcitonin or the response of the calcitonin level to a standard calcium stimulus can be assessed.

Men have higher circulating calcitonin levels than women and with age there is a fall in the response of calcitonin to calcium stimulation. Calcitonin levels increase with pregnancy, lactation and oestrogen replacement therapy and following alcohol consumption. A fall in calcitonin may accompany loss of ovarian function. Neither the total absence of calcitonin, as in thyroidectomy, nor overproduction of calcitonin, as in medullary thyroid cancer, produce much effect on the skeleton. The doses of calcitonin used therapeutically are higher than those provided by intrinsic secretion.

Calcitonin treatment

Epidemiological data suggest that calcitonin may reduce the risk of hip fractures,[8] but there have been few properly controlled long-term studies of calcitonin therapy in osteoporosis using reduction in fracture rate as the outcome measure. Salmon calcitonin has been most studied. Synthetic analogues of eel calcitonin are available. Genetically engineered human calcitonin is available but less effective. Compliance with treatment by injection is not high but salmon and eel analogues of calcitonin, available as nasal sprays, can be absorbed through the nasal mucosa, and are well tolerated.

The inhibitory effect of calcitonins on osteoclastic bone resorption is demonstrated by their effectiveness in Paget's disease and the acute

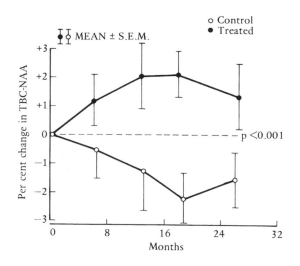

Figure 9.1   The effect of salmon calcitonin on total body calcium content (TBC) measured by neutron activation analysis (NAA).

The use of synthetic salmon calcitonin for the treatment of postmenopausal osteoporosis is approved by the Federal Drugs Administration in the USA and by the Medicines Control Agency in the UK. The dosage recommended varies from 50 IU units three times a week with oral calcium supplements, to 100 or 200 IU given for five days a week, which may be more effective. When treatment is stopped bone loss recurs.

Calcitonin has been shown to relieve spinal bone pain associated with osteoporosis in a controlled trial against placebo as measured by the number of analgesic tablets required.[26]

Adverse effects of calcitonin are few. Flushing following injection, which may last for up to two hours, is troublesome in one-quarter of patients but can often be prevented by pizotifen or cyproheptadine. A bonus of calcitonin is the relief of bone pain, and a disadvantage is the expense and inconvenience if used parenterally.

bone loss associated with immobility. Salmon calcitonin has been found to be effective in preventing the bone resorption which accompanies paraplegia in traumatic spinal cord injury.[21] In an early study of established osteoporosis, Chesnut et al.[22] randomly allocated 24 out of 50 patients to treatment with 100 MRC units of salmon calcitonin daily for 25–29 months. The controls and the treated patients also received 1200 mg of calcium carbonate and 400 IU of vitamin D daily. There was an increase in total body calcium as judged by neutron activation analysis (see Figure 9.1), which contrasted with a loss in the controls.

In women who were not more than three years postmenopausal, nasal calcitonin plus calcium resulted in a nonsignificant rise in bone density while control women treated with calcium lost a significant amount of bone.[23,24] In a study of women with osteoporosis aged 68–72 years,[25] in comparison with calcium, nasal calcitonin reduced the rates of fracture by two-thirds and increased their spinal bone masses in a dose-dependent manner.

BISPHOSPHONATES

Bisphosphonates are powerful inhibitors of osteoclastic activity and prevent bone resorption. They bind to the bone mineral crystals. Many bisphosphonates have been synthesized. Etidronate, the earliest to be marketed, can show seven years of successful suppression of bone loss and secondary prevention of spinal fractures in women. Bisphosphonates are similar in structure to pyrophosphate but the P–O–P bond is replaced by a P–C–P bond, leading to greater stability and resistance to enzymatic destruction (see Figure 9.2). They have a strong avidity for calcium ions, are rapidly taken up by bone and have a long skeletal half-life. They are very poorly absorbed and this is affected by any food or calcium-containing liquids, even mineral water or black coffee.

They inhibit crystal formation, aggregation and dissolution. This can lead to mineralization defects, which can result in osteomalacia. It is a physicochemical effect, reversible and is dose-

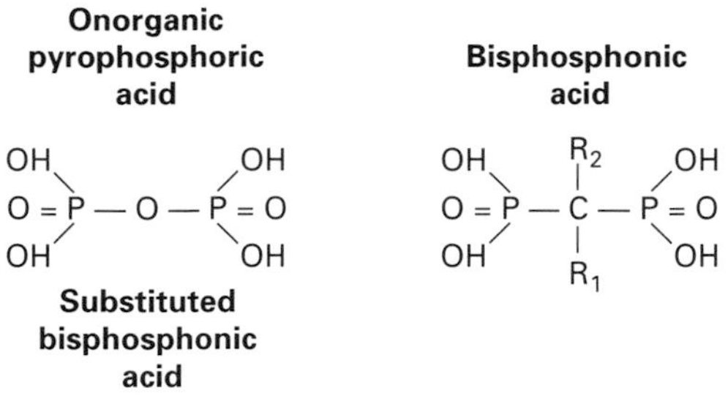

Onorganic pyrophosphoric acid	Bisphosphonic acid

$$O = P - O - P = O$$

with OH groups

$$O = P - C - P = O$$

with R_2, R_1 and OH groups

Substituted bisphosphonic acid

Compound	R_1	R_2
Etidronate	–OH	–CH$_3$
Pamidronate	–OH	–(CH2)$_2$–NH$_2$
Alendronate	–OH	–(CH2)$_3$–NH$_2$
Neridronate	–OH	–(CH2)$_5$–NH$_2$
Ibandronate	–OH	–(CH2)$_2$–N–CH$_3$.(CH$_2$)$_4$–CH$_3$
Clodronate	–Cl	–Cl
Tiludronate	–H	–S– –Cl
Risedronate	OH	–CH$_2$

Figure 9.2 Structure of bisphosphonates.

dependent. In clinical use only the doses of etidronate are high enough to have this effect, although in practice it does not appear to be a problem. The important action of bisphosphonates that is relevant to the treatment of osteoporosis, and to other conditions such as Paget's disease and hypercalcaemia, is the inhibition of bone resorption. The mechanism of this action is not yet clear. Their potency with respect to bone resorption varies. The doses at which they impair bone resorption and mineralization are close for etidronate but well separated for tiludronate, clodronate, pamidronate, alendronate and other more recent agents. These potencies are dependent on the side-chains and differ by over a thousandfold.

Controlled trials of bisphosphonates, in which the main outcome measure is fracture prevention, are technically difficult, take several years and involve large numbers of subjects. There are fewer problems when the outcome measure is prevention of loss of bone mass. Reduction of the rate of bone loss in osteoporotic women has been shown for etidronate, pamidronate, alendronate, clodronate, tiludronate, ibandronate and risedronate. Two randomly allocated controlled trials of a cyclical regime of etidronate have also confirmed prevention of further spinal fractures in postmenopausal osteoporotic women. These used two weeks of etidronate sodium 400 mg/day plus calcium followed by calcium citrate 500 mg for 11 weeks, the cycle then being repeated.[27–29] Calcium and etidronate are not taken at the same time of day as they interact to form insoluble complexes.

Alendronate, given as 10 mg daily, has been shown to increase progressively the bone mass in the spine, hip and total body. It has also been shown to reduce the incidence of vertebral fractures, the progression of vertebral deformities and the loss of height in postmenopausal women with osteoporosis and, additionally, alendronate can reduce the risk of limb fractures[30,31] (see Figure 9.3). Non-compliance with oral alendronate is about 30% after six months, mainly because of oesophageal and gastrointestinal irritation. Ibandronate given intravenously every three months for 12 months in a placebo controlled trial resulted in a significant dose-related improvement in spinal bone density in postmenopausal women. Improvement was also seen in the femoral neck. Compliance, often a problem with oral bisphosphonates, is predicted to be high when the drug is released for general prescription.[32]

Bisphosphonates are effective in preventing steroid-induced bone loss and there is more data available for cyclical etidronate.[33]

Toxicity and interactions[28]

The toxicity of etidronate is low but includes occasional hypersensitivity reactions. Etidronate and probably other bisphosphonates can worsen symptoms in osteomalacia. Pamidronate given intravenously may cause transient fever and leucopenia, and increases in bone pain. One patient with Paget's disease has

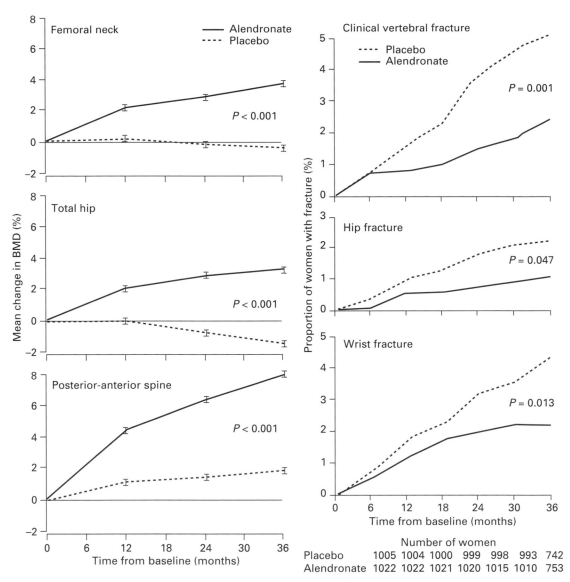

Mean percentage changes in BMD from baseline in women receiving alendronate or placebo for 36 months. Error bars, SE; BMD, bone mineral density.

Cumulative proportions of women with clinical vertebral fracture, hip fracture, or wrist fracture

Figure 9.3   The effect of alendronate on bone density and fracture. An increase in bone density is paralleled by a reduction in fractures.[31] Reproduced with permission from The Lancet Ltd (Black DM, Cummings SR, Karpf DB et al (1996) Randomised trial of effect of alendronate on risk of fracture in women with existing vertebral fractures. *Lancet* **348**: 1535–41).

been reported to develop recurrent iritis first with risedronate and later when challenged with pamidronate. Larger doses of pamidronate have caused visual hallucinations. Bisphosphonates interact with iron and magnesium treatments and should be separated from them by at least four hours. Alendronate shows effectiveness plus low toxicity provided that it is taken according to the recommended instructions.[31] These are that the drug should be taken on an empty stomach with at least half a glass of water and the subject should not sit down for half an hour. These instructions are onerous for elderly people. They are designed to stop the tablet lodging in the oesophagus. A significant proportion of spinal osteoporosis sufferers have a hiatus hernia, and many elderly people forget or disregard their instructions. Oesophagitis and even oesophageal stricture has been reported with alendronate when the instructions have not been followed. Risedronate and ibandronate are at earlier stages of development. Tiludronate is currently prescribable only for Paget's disease, and pamidronate and clodronate only for Paget's disease and tumoural hypercalcaemia in the UK.

All bisphosphonates are inactivated if taken with a meal. The avidity of some of the newer bisphosphonates such as ibandronate for calcium is such that they are best given parenterally in case the ionized calcium in the gastric and intestinal secretions inactivates them. Some bisphosphonates still under development are 500 to 3000 times more powerful than etidronate and different approaches to delivery, such as percutaneous, are being examined that promise to increase compliance.

Bisphosphonates interact with tetracyclines and should not be given together. The drugs are renally excreted and precautions are needed in chronic renal disease.

Bisphosphonates have been used in children with idiopathic juvenile osteoporosis with apparent reduction in fracture rate, but controlled trials are not available. Caution is needed because of the possible effects on skeletal growth. Bisphosphonates do not seem to impede fracture healing and there is no

evidence as yet of long-term toxicity if recommended regimes of treatment and dosage are given. However, bisphosphonates bind to hydroxyapatite crystals, seemingly irreversibly, and it may be years before attributable toxicity will show up and be recognized.

ANABOLIC STEROIDS

The anabolic steroids are synthetic derivatives of testosterone developed so as to increase anabolic activity and minimize androgenic effects. Of those studied (methandrostenolone, stanozolol and nandrolone decanoate) only the last is currently available. Anabolic steroids can rebuild bone in both men and women but their usefulness is limited by their adverse effects. In women, there is a tendency to deepening of the voice, which does not change when treatment is stopped, as well as the growth of facial hair. In men, there is the possibility of suppression of normal gonadal function. Since anabolic steroids are 17-methylated heterocyclic steroids they produce liver function abnormalities with frequent elevation of the serum aspartate aminotransferase and occasionally elevation of serum alkaline phosphatase and bilirubin levels. Other potentially serious adverse effects include hepatoma (associated with higher doses), elevation of low density lipoproteins and reduction of high density lipoprotein plasma concentrations, which might predispose to ischaemic heart disease.

It seems wise to limit the use of an anabolic steroid to short-term prescription to take advantage of the well recognized effect in limiting post-traumatic loss of nitrogen and calcium. Giving nandrolone decanoate in oil by a single injection of 50 mg once a week for three weeks in the aftermath of a spinal fracture may shorten the period of convalescence and pain. The evidence for this is anecdotal but it is difficult to see how evidence from a controlled trial could be obtained, given the unpredictability of such episodes and the variability of the natural course of episodes of spinal fracture.

VITAMIN D

Vitamin D activity is essential for the normal development of the skeleton, as mineralization of osteoid and absorption of calcium from the gut are controlled by vitamin D metabolites. Although originally considered to be a vitamin, it is now classed as a hormone, as 90% of bodily needs for vitamin D are supplied in the skin by the conversion by ultraviolet light of 7-dehydrocholesterol to vitamin D_3 (cholecalciferol). Cholecalciferol is biologically inactive until it has been converted to hydroxycholecalciferol (25-hydroxy-vitamin D) in the liver. 25-Hydroxy-vitamin D circulates in the blood and the level there is taken as the best measure of vitamin D status. Further hydroxylation of 25-hydroxy-vitamin D in the kidney leads to 1,25-dihydroxy-vitamin D_3 (calcitriol), the biologically active end product. Dermal synthesis of vitamin D_3 is fail-safe in that dermally made vitamin D_3 is itself subjected to photodegradation from various photometabolites, and sunlight does not produce vitamin D toxicity except in those who suffer from sarcoidosis. Complete deprivation of sunlight, even in young men on a normal diet, is followed within three months by halving of blood levels of 25-hydroxy-vitamin D and doubling of faecal calcium losses and a negative calcium balance.[34] Vitamin D_2, ergocalciferol, is made by the action of ultraviolet light on the fungal steroid, ergosterol, and follows the same metabolic pathway. The chief dietary sources of vitamin D are fish and fish oils. In contrast to dermal synthesis, excessive amounts of prescribed vitamin D are toxic and can cause net loss of bone, hypercalciuria and hypercalcaemia. Vitamin D made or absorbed in the summer is stored in the body for the winter in high latitudes where the winter sun does not rise high enough for ultraviolet rays to penetrate atmospheric moisture. Also possibly linked to sunlight exposure, there is a north/south gradient for osteoporotic hip fracture. There is a similar north/south gradient for coronary heart disease which, it has been suggested, is due to wintertime diversion of squalene metabolism to cholesterol rather than vitamin D synthesis.[35]

Vitamin D in the elderly

Elderly people are less able than the young to synthesize vitamin D in the skin from a given flux of ultraviolet light.[36] Calcium absorption also falls with age, as do 25-hydroxy-vitamin D levels, mainly due to lack of exposure to sunlight and poor diet.[37] 1,25-Dihydroxy-vitamin D_3 levels are low or normal in postmenopausal osteoporosis. It remains unclear whether the low calcium absorption seen in elderly people arises from the low levels of 1,25-dihydroxy-vitamin D_3 synthesis or intake, or from resistance of the gut to its actions, or whether it is a combination of these factors. Recent evidence suggests that in some elderly osteoporotic female patients there can be relative resistance to vitamin D; 500–1000 IU daily having no effect over a six-month period when alfacalcidol 0.25 µg twice daily was effective in increasing calcium absorption.[38]

Thus, vitamin D, 1,25-dihydroxy-vitamin D_3 (calcitriol) and 1-α-vitamin D (alfacalcidol) improve calcium absorption in osteoporotic and nonosteoporotic subjects. However, if the body is already vitamin D replete they will also increase plasma and urine calcium and will not have a positive effect on calcium balance,[39] nor reduce the rates of loss of cortical bone mass or of deterioration of vertebral morphometry in established osteoporosis.

More recent studies, noting that average vitamin D intake has declined in the last 30 years in Britain, have shown a positive correlation between vitamin D blood levels and bone density and a negative correlation with intact parathyroid hormone concentrations.[40] Moreover, some elderly patients with apparent osteoporotic femoral neck fracture have been shown to have histological evidence of

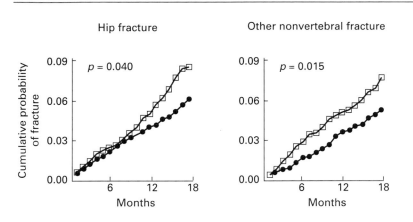

Figure 9.4 Hip and other nonvertebral fractures in elderly institutionalized women treated either with 800 IU vitamin D_3 and 1200 mg elemental calcium or with placebo.[43] Placebo group, □; vitamin D_3 and calcium group, ●. Estimated by the Life-Table Method and based on the length of time to the first fracture.

osteomalacia[41] as have those who suffer from rheumatoid arthritis.[42]

Vitamin D supplementation has been studied in institutionalized elderly women in France, with a mean age of 84 years.[43,44] A controlled comparison of vitamin D_3 800 IU plus calcium supplementation of 1200 mg compared with placebo over three years resulted in 29% fewer hip fractures and the total number of nonspinal fractures was 24% lower, even in the absence of conventional criteria for osteomalacia. There were significantly less fractures within 18 months (see Figure 9.4). In contrast, a study of elderly (mean age 80 years), but mainly independent men and women living in The Netherlands[45] found no prevention of nonspinal fractures with vitamin D_3 400 IU/day compared with placebo over a maximum of three and a half years on a background of a higher calcium intake. These results are interpreted as showing that supplementing calcium and vitamin D_3 in the frail elderly who live indoors and who are deficient in both will prevent fractures. This is supported by the reduction in PTH secretion in the French institutionalized women who received vitamin D and who were shown to have increased their vitamin D levels.[43] Increasing the vitamin D blood level in those who are depleted will reduce the PTH drive to mobilize calcium from the skeleton.

What has become clear is that depletion of vitamin D is increasingly common in the elderly or the disabled for a variety of reasons. The only safe criterion for depletion is a low blood level of 25-hydroxy-vitamin D. The presence of widened osteoid seams on histology of bone biopsy, usually taken as the signature of osteomalacia and hence of vitamin D depletion, is not applicable to most elderly people. The reciprocal relationship between vitamin D and PTH levels was exemplified by the French study[43] and an elevated PTH is an indicator of vitamin D deficiency.

These studies show that deficiency should be avoided, but that giving vitamin D supplementation to those who are already vitamin D replete would not do any good. Where facilities exist for its measurement, the aim should be to raise the blood level of 25-hydroxy-vitamin D to between 20 and 80 nmol/l. This can be achieved by 400–800 IU of vitamin D daily or by giving a single oral dose of 100 000 IU of vitamin D_3 each winter. In summer, some daily exposure of the hands, forearms and lower legs to sunlight should be arranged when weather permits. Installing broad-spectrum fluorescent lights which emit a small amount of ultraviolet light, and substituting polycarbonate glazing in conservatories in old people's homes, should have the same results, but cost benefit calculations have not been done on these various measures. They should be favourable if only a few hip fractures are prevented because of the high cost of hip replacement arthroplasty or other surgical treatment.

VITAMIN D METABOLITES

Calcitriol (1,25-dihydroxy-vitamin D_3) is the most active metabolite of vitamin D, and alfacalcidol (1α-hydroxy-vitamin D) is a synthetic analogue. There have been several studies of these metabolites with variable results. A large controlled trial examined calcitriol in women in New Zealand with a mean age of 64 years who had sustained vertebral fracture. In a single blind study they compared calcitriol 0.5 µg/day with calcium 1 g/day over three years and found fewer new vertebral fractures in the calcitriol group.[46] Curiously, the difference was due to the rate of new vertebral fractures staying stable in the group receiving calcitriol but increasing in the calcium group. The role of these metabolites in preventing further osteoporotic fractures has not been clearly established.

PARATHYROID HORMONE (PTH)

Parathyroid hormone maintains the extracellular fluid calcium concentration, acting directly on the kidney and bone. It stimulates renal synthesis of 1,25-dihydroxy-vitamin D_3, which increases intestinal absorption of calcium. It also stimulates bone formation, probably by the activation of the basic multicellular units (BMUs) of bone. The 1–34 aminoterminal fragment of this 84-amino acid polypeptide is the active component which has been most often prescribed. Fragments less than 1–32 lose activity on bone cells. Fragment 1–34 of human PTH (hPTH[1–34]) has been synthesized and a multicentre study has shown its effectiveness in established osteoporosis.[47] Sixteen patients were treated with 50–100 µg of human PTH as a daily subcutaneous injection for six months. There was an increase in trabecular bone volume with the formation of new bone on the surface of existing trabeculae, but there was no improvement in calcium balance nor in cortical bone density. This suggested that the increase in trabecular bone might be at the expense of cortical bone. Subsequent studies have generally used lower dose levels (25–40 µg) in combination with antiresorptive agents such as oestrogen, calcitonin or a bisphosphonate. Most recently, in a three-year randomized study of 34 osteoporotic women with a stable bone density on HRT, half of the women received 400 IU/25 µg daily subcutaneously.[48] There was a 13% increase in vertebral bone density in those treated with the PTH peptide compared with an insignificant fall in those on HRT alone. Most of the increase in vertebral bone density was in the first year, with an increase in osteocalcin within one month and in N-telopeptide levels over six months, and both then returning to baseline. Smaller increases in bone density were noted at the hip. There were fewer new vertebral deformities in those receiving hPTH[1–34], but a larger study would be necessary to prove fracture prevention.

ANDROGENS

Ten per cent of men with osteoporosis have low circulating androgen levels. If the comparison is limited to elderly men with hip fracture this rises to over 50%, a 4.6 times increase compared with case controls.[49] In some, but not all, instances this responds to testosterone treatment.

In postmenopausal women, testosterone has been used as co-therapy with oestradiol implants. The addition appears to make little difference to the effectiveness in protecting bone but improves libido and probably compliance with repeat implants.

SELECTIVE ESTROGEN RECEPTOR MODULATORS

Selective Estrogen Receptor Modulators (SERMS) is the name given for a class of drugs which are tissue-specific and block oestrogen receptors in breast tissue, but act as a pro-oestrogen in bone. How they exert their tissue-selective effects is unclear but will be better understood as the multiple molecular pathways that are involved in mediating oestrogen activity are identified. Tamoxifen is the best known of these and studies have shown a small effect of tamoxifen on vertebral bone mass. Raloxifene and droloxifene share the favourable actions of tamoxifen on bones, breasts and cardiovascular system, but differ in being inhibitory to the endometrium.[50] Raloxifene improves bone density and the serum lipid profile in ovarectomised rats but has little oestrogenic activity on breast and uterine tissues. In a randomised placebo-controlled dose-ranging study, raloxifene given for two years to post-menopausal women resulted in a significant increase in spine and hip bone mineral density, with a similar benefit to cortical and trabecular bone.[51] There was no increase in endothelial thickness and serum total cholesterol and low-density lipoprotein cholesterol did not change. Raloxifene is approved by the FDA for the prevention of osteoporosis in postmenopausal women.

OTHER AGENTS

Phytoestrogens

Plant isoflavones and lignans with antioxidant and phytoestrogenic properties are widespread in vegetables and fruits. Some have weak anticancer properties. Soya protein, which is rich in the isoflavone phytoestrogen genistein, forms a considerable part of the diet of women in Asia. Asian women are reported to have menstrual periods lasting two days longer than western women and they have half the incidence of breast cancer. Cassidy et al.,[52] in a study using western women as their own controls, showed that a diet high in soya protein increased the follicular phase of the menstrual cycle and suppressed LH and FSH levels. It was suggested that genistein was tamoxifen-like, i.e., blocking oestrogen receptors in the breast but having oestrogen-like effects on receptors in bone and vascular tissue.[52] Proof of this awaits further studies.

The drug ipriflavone[53,54] is derived from soya isoflavone. It has weak phytoestrogen properties. It is effective in preserving bone density in early postmenopausal osteoporosis and increases bone density at the radius and lumbar spine in established osteoporosis. There is little data as yet on fracture prevention. It is licensed in some countries.

Strontium

Strontium is the element most closely related to calcium and it follows calcium metabolic pathways in the body. It is not thought to be an essential trace element. Preliminary evidence suggests that low dose strontium supplements increase bone formation and decrease bone resorption, and may be unique in that it can uncouple bone formation and resorption.[54] Clinical studies have been encouraging with strontium ranelate (S-12911), a divalent strontium salt.[55]

Zeolite-A

Silicon appears to be an essential trace element. Uncontrolled trials suggest that silano-salicylate increases bone strength. Zeolite-A is a silicon compound given to hens to increase eggshell hardness and the strength of bones, and which has been tendered as worth testing in human osteoporosis.

Boron

Boron is an essential trace element. Deficiency leads to bone weakness which can be corrected by giving boron. Despite efforts to promote boron in proprietary medicines as a treatment for osteoporosis, no convincing human studies have been published.

Others

Vitamin K is involved in the production of osteocalcin. Circulating vitamin K levels are depressed in osteoporotic subjects. It has been suggested that increased bone marrow fat in elderly people may sequester fat-soluble vitamins and make them less available to osteoblasts. Clinical trials have not been done except as part of a general improvement in the diet of elderly people, which improves the prognosis in osteoporosis.

Growth hormone increases markers of bone formation and bone density in growth hormone-deficient subjects. The action is thought to be mediated by insulin-like growth factors. So far, neither have found a place in treating disorders of bone other than those caused by deficiency.

Thiazide diuretics reduce the urinary loss of calcium. The effect appears to be temporary but could be important in conjunction with measures to increase calcium deposition in bone.

LIFESTYLE

The importance of lifestyle has already been discussed as a means of prevention (see Chapter 7). There are no specific data on the effect of reducing alcohol consumption or smoking for those with osteoporosis. Moderate alcohol intake is associated with a small increase in bone density. Excess alcohol is, however, associated with reduced bone density, more falls and fractures. Smoking is associated with reduced bone density and increased risk of fracture. Ex-smokers have a similar bone density as nonsmokers.[56]

Exercise

Patients also need to be counselled on exercise. It is beneficial at any age, although the benefits are greater in younger subjects. Weight-bearing exercise, such as walking, is superior to swimming but the latter is useful in the rehabilitation of patients after surgery for limb fracture or episodes of spinal crush fracture. Exercise not only improves bone density, it strengthens muscles and improves postural stability, and hence has a role in preventing falls. People with lesser degrees of osteoporosis should be encouraged to undertake social and physical activities which provide exercise such as dancing, gardening, carpentry or walking the dog.

FALL PREVENTION

Once osteoporotic, the main discriminator as to who will fracture and who will not is sustaining a fall. Preventing falls or reducing the impact of a fall are therefore important strategies in reducing the risk of fracture. The physically weak are at most risk and approaches that have been used with variable results have been exercise programmes, balance training, and home assessments to identify and correct intrinsic and extrinsic risk factors such as inappropriate drug therapy or hazards such as loose rugs.[57] It is important to try but difficult to achieve fall prevention and another approach is to reduce the impact of a fall with hip protectors, which have been shown to be effective in preventing fracture amongst nursing home residents.[58] The relative risk of hip fracture amongst those wearing a protector was 0.44. It is unclear how effective they are in the setting of nursing homes and own homes outside a research protocol, when compliance is the greater issue.

PAIN CONTROL IN OSTEOPOROSIS

Uncomplicated osteoporosis, simple loss of bone density, is not painful. So why do some osteoporosis sufferers complain of pain? There are no pain nerve endings in bone itself. In contrast, the periosteum and the attachments of ligaments and tendons (entheses) are rich in pain nerve endings and there are nonmedullated pain fibres which accompany blood vessels within bones.

One of the mysteries of osteoporosis is that a patient can present with multiple spinal crush fractures yet complain only of loss of height. Presumably their spinal shrinkage reflects the sum of many small episodes of trabecular fractures and remodelling, no one episode being severe enough to breach the pain threshold. But in other sufferers, spinal pain can be severe and enduring. Several possible mechanisms present themselves for consideration.

Pain in a bone can arise from changes in intraosseous pressure. Thus, in sternal bone marrow aspiration quite severe pain may occur as the plunger of the syringe is withdrawn, even if the skin and periosteum have been fully anaesthetized. Rises of intraosseous pressure associated with abnormalities of venous run-off have been demonstrated in painful osteoarthritis and aseptic necrosis of the femoral head. More obviously, since it can sometimes be visualized on X-ray, pain is related to intraosseous bleeding and haematoma. The various causes of regional osteoporosis are often painful, with the pain arising from the intraosseous hyperaemia, as in the osteoporotic forms of Paget's disease.

Pain in the acute spinal crush fracture syndrome, as described in Chapter 6, is generally self-limiting as the fracture heals. But such fractures should always be investigated both to rule out other causes of vertebral collapse (such as hyperparathyroidism, multiple myelomatosis and spinal metastases) and also to detect often treatable underlying predisposing causes of osteoporosis such as thyrotoxicosis, Cushing's syndrome and gonadal failure. Enduring pain in spinal shrinkage is usually ascribed to the consequent stresses on the apophyseal joints and spinal ligaments. There is also the possibility that it may be caused by obstruction of the veins entering the spinal canal through the neural foramina, causing oedema and fibrosis of the nerve roots. However, clinicians will recognize, particularly when no analgesics seem to work, that in some instances it is a 'cry for help' from a lonely and disabled elderly person. If 'morphine is no better than an aspirin' use aspirin and look for underlying social distress.

Secondary neck pain and tension headaches may be caused by the difficulty of holding the head up because of thoracic kyphosis, and lumbar spinal shrinkage may cause painful impaction of the lower ribs on the pelvic brim.

Unless these underlying causes of pain are considered, opportunities to help will be missed. In particular it is wrong, as is unfortunately often the case when patients in pain are found to have low bone density on scanning, to say 'You have osteoporosis' as though that were a sufficient explanation.

The severity of pain of the acute vertebral fracture should not be underestimated and opiates may be necessary in the short term to achieve pain control. Where specific treatments are unavailable, it is worth trying a course of calcitonin injections due to their reported actions in reducing bone pain, or a bisphosphonate such as alendronate for painful regional osteoporosis. Otherwise, the control of pain is similar to that in other painful conditions.

It is important to remember that pain control is often not achieved because the patient for various reasons decides to ration their use of simple analgesics for fear of 'hurting themselves whilst masking the pain', 'getting used to them' or fear of side-effects. Educating the patient overcomes this.

SURGERY AND SPLINTING

For spinal osteoporosis, spinal supports are required only rarely. When they are, it is almost always in patients with extremely severe osteoporosis, such as those on obligatory long-term corticosteroid therapy. Short lumbosacral corsets to help relieve back pain can be worn by some patients but not if abdominal distension due to shrinkage of the lumbar spine has reduced the capacity of the abdominal cavity.

Surgery for osteoporosis other than that which is required for the mending of fractures is still tentative and experimental. Osteotomies of the lumbar spine and lower cervical spine may rarely be needed when there is severe flexion deformity at these levels. As spinal shrinkage often involves the lower thoracic spine, osteotomy at that level is not practical. Pain relief in thoracic spinal collapse has been reported from procedures which stiffen the trabeculae of vertebral bodies by injecting a biocompatible cement. Occasionally, the lower ribs may need to be removed if they impact painfully on the pelvic margin. A troublesome hiatus hernia or pelvic floor impairment with rectal or uterine prolapse may need to be treated surgically. Sometimes, prism glasses are needed for patients so bent that they have difficulty in seeing forwards when walking. A portable foam cushion with carrying handle is useful in raising seat heights whilst driving, eating out, or going to a theatre. For thin, and usually institutionalized, elderly patients, special padded hip protectors have been designed (see page 189). Several models are now available. Their effectiveness in preventing hip fracture has been demonstrated in a controlled clinical trial.[58]

COUNSELLING

As with any long-term treatment proper management and counselling are essential for good compliance and time must be set aside for this, as many women conceal worries unless encouraged to reveal them. A good start to a counselling interview is, 'Tell me what you know about hormone replacement therapy—I don't want to tell you what you already know.' This will encourage the patient to set out her own ideas which can be improved upon or modified as necessary. Fears such as the return of 'mini-periods' might mean to the patient that fertility will return. Worries about breast cancer need to be discussed. The value of exercise and of a diet delivering adequate calcium need to be ventilated. Many patients become frightened to go out because of their 'fragile skeletons'. A comprehensive osteoporosis service will include a telephone helpline. Regular follow-up needs to be organized if compliance is to be for years rather than months

SELF-HELP SOCIETIES

These have been and are being established in various countries. In the UK, the National Osteoporosis Society (Charity No. 292660; address: PO Box 10, Radstock, Bath BA3 3YB) publishes a newsletter where shared concerns can be aired (issues such as genetic inheritance, practical problems with driving, tailoring, etc.) and where news of research endeavours into the cause, prevention and treatment of osteoporosis can be reported in lay language. An educational publication, *Osteoporosis Review*, informs health professionals about relevant topics and current research papers.

In the USA, there is the National Osteoporosis Foundation (address: 1625 Eye Street NW, Suite 1011, Washington, DC 20006).

The Board of National Societies of the European Foundation for Osteoporosis can supply names and addresses of member organizations in Europe (Secretary: Professor Peter Burkhardt, Department of Internal Medicine, CHUV, CH-1011 Lausanne, Switzerland).

PRACTICAL POINTS

Recommendations for treatment

Before treatment confirm the diagnosis

In order to rule out other conditions with 'thin' bones on X-ray or where there has been a fracture after minimal trauma.
* Blood
  —full blood count, ESR or viscosity
  —serum calcium, phosphate and alkaline phosphatase
  —serum and urine electrophoresis if suspicious of myeloma
  —thyroid function
  —serum testosterone in men
* X-ray
  —to confirm vertebral fracture
* Bone densitometry
* Bone biopsy if necessary

Before treatment eliminate causes

* In rheumatoid arthritis and neurological conditions, improve mobility by pain control, physiotherapy and rehabilitation.
* In glucocorticoid-treated patients, keep long-term glucocorticoid dosage as low as possible. Consider the use of glucocorticoid-sparing agents such as azathioprine or methotrexate, use local or topical preparations wherever possible (i.e., intra-articular long-acting glucocorticoids in arthritis; inhalations of beclomethasone or similar in obstructive airways disease; low dose glucocorticoid ointment in skin diseases). Where systemic glucocorticoid treatment is unavoidable, consider switching to deflazacort or co-therapy with a bisphosphonate such as cyclical etidronate.
* In thyrotoxicosis treat the endocrine abnormality.
* In thyroid hormone overdosage gradually withdraw.
* Where possible correct other predisposing causes, such as smoking or lack of dietary calcium. If necessary, call in a dietician for assessment of current calcium intake.

In postmenopausal osteoporosis

* Give lifestyle and dietary advice and calcium supplements to bring the total calcium intake up to 1000–1500 mg daily. In the elderly or disabled, consider low dose vitamin D.
* Consider hormone replacement therapy using a cyclical low dose oestrogen–progestogen sequence, having warned the patient of the possibility of cyclical mastalgia and mini-periods. If these possibilities are likely to reduce compliance, consider a 'continuous-combined' form of HRT.
* Consider testosterone replacement in hypogonadal men with osteoporosis.
* For osteoporotic women who do not accept HRT and for osteoporotic men who are eugonadal, consider treatment with a bisphosphonate, calcitonin or calcitriol.

REFERENCES

1. Matkovic V, Kostial K, Simonovic I et al. Bone status and fracture rates in two regions of Yugoslavia. *Am J Clin Nutr* (1974), **32**: 361–3.
2. Holbrook TL, Barrett-Connor E, Wingard DL. Dietary calcium and risk of hip fracture: 14-year prospective population study. *Lancet* (1988), ii: 1046–9.
3. Heaney RP, Recker RR, Saville PD. Calcium balance and calcium requirements in middle-aged women. *Am J Clin Nutr* (1977), **30**: 1603–11.
4. Riis B, Thomsen K, Christiansen C. Does calcium supplementation prevent postmenopausal bone loss? *N Engl J Med* (1987), **316**: 173–7.
5. Dawson-Hughes B, Dallal GE, Krall EA et al. A controlled trial of the effect of calcium supplementation on bone density in postmenopausal women. *N Engl J Med* (1990), **323**: 878–83.
6. Prince RL, Smith M, Dick IM et al. Prevention of postmenopausal osteoporosis. *N Engl J Med* (1991), **325**: 1189–95.
7. Reid IR, Ames RW, Evans MC et al. Effects of calcium supplementation in postmenopausal women. *N Engl J Med* (1993), **328**: 460–4.
8. Kanis JA, Johnell O, Gullberg B et al. Evidence of efficacy of drugs affecting bone metabolism in preventing hip fracture. *Br Med J* (1992), **305**: 1124–8.
9. Recker RR, Hinders S, Davies KM et al. Correcting calcium nutritional deficiency prevents spine fractures in elderly women. *J Bone Miner Res* (1996), **11**: 1961–6.
10. Dawson-Hughes B, Harris SS, Krall EA et al. Effect of calcium and vitamin D supplementation on bone density in men and women 65 years of age or older. *New Engl J Med* (1997) **337**: 701–2.
11. Cumming RG, Nevitt MC. Calcium for prevention of osteoporotic fractures in postmenopausal women. *J Bone Min Res* (1997) **12**: 1321–9.
12. Epstein O, Kato Y, Dick R et al. Vitamin D, hydroxyapatite and calcium gluconate in treatment of cortical bone thinning in postmenopausal women with primary biliary cirrhosis. *Am J Clin Nutr* (1982), **36**: 426–30.
13. Nilson KH, Jayson MIV, Dixon A St J. Microcrystalline hydroxyapatite compound in corticosteroid-treated rheumatoid patients, a controlled study. *Br Med J* (1978), **2**: 1124–6.
14. Reid IR, Ibbotson HK. Calcium supplements in steroid-induced osteoporosis. *Am J Clin Nutr* (1986), **44**: 287–90.
15. Bernstein DS, Sadowsky N, Hegstead DM et al. Prevalence of osteoporosis in high- and low-fluoride areas of North Dakota. *JAMA* (1966), **198**: 499–504.
16. Moller PF, Gudjonsson SV. Massive fluorosis of bones and ligaments. *Acta Radiol* (1932), **13**: 269–94.
17. Gordon SL, Corbin SB. Summary of workshop on drinking water fluoride influence on hip fracture on bone health, National Institutes of Health, 10 April 1991. *Osteoporos Int* (1992), **2**: 109–17.
18. Hedlund LR, Gallagher JC. Increased incidence of hip fracture in osteoporotic women treated with sodium fluoride. *J Bone Miner Res* (1989), **4**: 223–7.
19. Riggs BL, Hodgson SF, O'Fallon WM et al. Effect of fluoride treatment on the fracture rate in postmenopausal women with osteoporosis. *N Engl J Med* (1990), **322**: 802–9.
20. Mamelle N, Dusan R, Meunier DJ et al. Risk–benefit ratio of sodium fluoride treatment in primary vertebral osteoporosis. *Lancet* (1988), ii: 361–5.
21. Minaire P et al. Treatment of acute osteoporosis due to paraplegia with calcitonin. *Clin Sci* (1982), **62**: 42.
22. Chesnut CH III, Sisom K, Nelp WB et al. Are synthetic salmon calcitonin and anabolic steroids efficacious in the treatment of postmenopausal osteoporosis? In: Dixon A St J et al. eds. *Osteoporosis, a multidisciplinary problem.* Academic Press: London (1983), pp. 239–44.
23. Reginster JY, Albert A, Lecart MP et al. 1-year controlled randomised trial of prevention of early postmenopausal bone loss by intranasal calcitonin. *Lancet* (1987), ii: 1481–3.
24. Reginster JY, Denis D, Deroisy R et al. Long-term (3 years) prevention of trabecular postmenopausal bone loss with low-dose intermittent nasal salmon calcitonin. *J Bone Miner Res* (1994), **9**: 69–73.
25. Overgaard K, Hansen MA, Jensen SB et al. Effect of salcatonin given intranasally on bone mass and fracture rates in established osteoporosis: a dose–response study. *Br Med J* (1992), **305**: 556–8.
26. Lyritis GP, Tsakalos N, Magiasis B et al. Analgesic effect of salmon calcitonin in osteoporotic vertebral fractures: a double-blind,

placebo controlled clinical study. *Calcif Tissue Int* (1991), **49**: 3679–82.

27. Storm T, Thamsborg G, Steiniche T et al. Effect of cyclical etidronate therapy on bone mass and fracture rate in women with postmenopausal osteoporosis. *N Engl J Med* (1990), **322**: 165–71.

28. Watts NH, Harris ST, Genant H et al. Intermittent cyclical treatment of postmenopausal osteoporosis. *N Engl J Med* (1990), **323**: 73–9.

29. Harris ST, Watts NB, Jackson RD et al. Four-year study of intermittent cyclic etidronate treatment of postmenopausal osteoporosis: three years of blinded therapy followed by one year of open therapy. *Am J Med* (1993), **95**: 557–67.

30. Libermann VA, Weiss SR, Broll J et al. Effect of oral alendronate on bone mineral density and the incidence of fractures in postmenopausal women. *N Engl J Med* (1995), **333**: 1437–43.

31. Black DM, Cummings SR, Karpf DB et al. Randomised trial of effect of alendronate on risk of fracture in women with existing vertebral fractures. *Lancet* (1996), **348**: 1535–41.

32. Thiébaud D, Burckhardt P, Kriegbaum J et al. Three-monthly injections of ibandronate in the treatment of postmenopausal osteoporosis. *Amer J Med* (1997) **13**: 298–307.

33. Adachi JD, Cranney A, Goldsmith CH et al. Intermittent cyclic therapy with etidronate in the prevention of corticosteroid induced bone loss. *J Rheumatol* (1994), **21**: 1922–6.

34. Davies DM. Calcium metabolism in healthy men deprived of sunlight. *Ann N Y Acad Sci* (1985), **453**: 21–7.

35. Grimes DS, Hindle E, Dyer T. Sunlight, cholesterol and coronary heart disease. *Q J Med* (1996), **89**: 579–89.

36. Maclaughlin A, Holick MF. Ageing decreases the capacity of human skin to produce vitamin D_3. *J Clin Invest* (1985), **76**: 1536–8.

37. van der Weilen RPJ, Lowick MRH, van den Berg H et al. Serum vitamin D concentrations among elderly people in Europe. *Lancet* (1995), **436**: 207–10.

38. Francis RM. Is there a differential response to alphacalcidol and vitamin-D in the treatment of osteoporosis? Communication no. SSu 021. *Osteoporos Int* (1996) **6**: (suppl. 1): 313.

39. Gallagher JC, Jerpbak CM, Jee WSS et al. 1,25-dihydroxy-vitamin D_3: short and long-term effects on calcium; metabolism in patients with postmenopausal osteoporosis. *Proc Natl Acad Sci U S A* (1982), **79**: 3325–9.

40. Khaw KT, Sneyd M-J, Compston J. Bone density, parathyroid hormone and 25-hydroxy-vitamin-D concentrations in middle-aged women. *Br Med J* (1992), **304**: 274–7.

41. Aaron JE, Gallagher JC, Anderson et al. Frequency of osteomalacia and osteoporosis in fractures of the proximal femur. *Lancet* (1974), **ii**: 84–5.

42. Ralston SH, Willcocks L, Pitkeathly DA et al. High prevalence of unrecognised osteomalacia in hospital patients with rheumatoid arthritis. *Br J Rheumatol* (1988), **27**: 202–5.

43. Chapuy MA, Arlot ME, Duboeuf F et al. Vitamin D_3 and calcium to prevent hip fractures in elderly women. *N Engl J Med* (1992), **327**: 1637–42.

44. Chapuy MA, Arlot ME, Delmas P et al. Effect of calcium and cholecalciferol treatment for three years on hip fractures in elderly women. *Br Med J* (1994), **308**: 1081–2.

45. Lips P, Graafmans WC, Ooms ME, Bezemer PD, Bouter LM. Vitamin D supplementation and fracture incidence in elderly persons. *Ann Intern Med* (1996), **124**: 400–6.

46. Tilyard M, Spears GFS, Thomson J et al. Treatment of postmenopausal osteoporosis with calcitriol or calcium. *N Engl J Med* (1992), **326**: 357–62.

47. Reeve J, Meunier PJ, Parsons JA et al. Anabolic effect of human parathyroid hormone fragment on trabecular bone in involutional osteoporosis: a multicentre trial. *Br Med J* (1980), **280**: 1340–4.

48. Lindsay R, Nieves J, Formica C et al. Randomised controlled study of effect of parathyroid hormone on vertebral-bone mass and fracture incidence among postmenopausal women on oestrogen with osteoporosis. *Lancet* (1997), **350**: 550–5.

49. Stanley HL, Schmitt BP, Poses RM et al. Does hypogonadism contribute to the occurrence of minimal hip trauma fracture in elderly men? *J Am Geriatr Soc* (1991), **39**: 766–71.

50. Draper MW, Flowers DE, Huster WJ et al. A controlled trial of raloxifene (LY139481) HCl: impact on bone turnover and serum lipid profile in healthy postmenopausal women. *J Bone Miner Res* (1996), **11**: 835–42.

51. Delmas P, Bjharnason N, Mitlak BH et al. Effects of raloxifene on bone mineral density, serum cholesterol concentrations and uterine endometrium in postmenopausal women. *New Engl J Med* (1997) **337**: 1641–7.

52. Cassidy A, Bingham S, Setchell KDR. Biological effects of a diet rich in isoflavones on the menstrual cycle of premenopausal women. *Am J Clin Nutr* (1994), **60**: 333–40.

53. Agnusdei D. Effect of ipriflavone in established osteoporosis and long-term safety. *Osteoporos Int* (1996), **6** (suppl 1): 318.

54. Marie PJ, Hott M, Modrowski D et al. An uncoupling agent containing strontium prevents bone loss by depressing bone resorption and maintaining bone formation in estrogen-deficient rats. *J Bone Miner Res* (1993), **8**: 607–15.

55. Meunier PJ, Slosman D, Delmas P et al. The strontium salt S 12911: a new candidate for the treatment of osteoporosis. *Osteoporos Int* (1996), **6** (suppl 1): 241.

56. Nguyen TV, Kelly PJ, Sambrook PN et al. Lifestyle factors and bone density in the elderly. *J Bone Miner Res* (1994), **9**: 1339–46.

57. Oakley A et al. Preventing falls and subsequent injury in older people. *Effective Health Care* (1996), **2**(4): 1–16.

58. Lauritzen JB, Petersen MM, Lund B. Effect of external hip protectors on hip fractures. *Lancet* (1993), **341**: 11–13.

Index